Amputated Lives
Coping with Chemical Sensitivity

Alison Johnson

With a Foreword by
L. Christine Oliver, M.D.
Harvard Medical School

Cumberland Press
Brunswick, Maine

Copyright © 2008 by Alison Johnson

Alison Johnson
Cumberland Press
Box 213
Brunswick, ME 04011

ISBN 13: 978-0-9675619-1-2

ISBN 10: 0-9675619-1-4

Printed in the United States of America

Amputated Lives
Coping with Chemical Sensitivity

Contents

Foreword

In her book *Amputated Lives: Coping with Chemical Sensitivity*, Alison Johnson brings to life a disease that affects millions of Americans. It is a disease that is not understood by physicians caring for these individuals. It is a disease that is not understood by employers. It is a disease not understood by family members. And perhaps most distressingly, it is a disease that is preventable. The name of this disease is chemical sensitivity, manifesting in its most severe form as multiple chemical sensitivity.

For those affected, this disease is often a prison sentence without parole. Homes can sometimes be made "safe." But environments outside the home cannot be controlled and therefore are not safe—tolerable maybe—but not safe. Chemical exposures occur unpredictably, with incapacitating consequences. These chemicals are ubiquitous and include perfumes, colognes, hair spray, detergents, carpet components, adhesives, pesticides, and vehicular exhaust.

It is no wonder that, as Johnson chronicles, individuals are disabled from work as a result of chemical sensitivity. Homes become uninhabitable, and alternative living arrangements are difficult to establish. Families are destroyed. At the very time when substantial economic resources are required to create a safe living environment, it is difficult for individuals with the disease to find a workplace that does not make them sick.

Chemical sensitivity makes every day a challenge for those affected. Chemical sensitivity also presents a challenge to physicians caring for these patients, as I have done for more than two decades as Co-Director of Occupational and Environmental Medicine at the Massachusetts General Hospital. For the physician, the first challenge is to make the diagnosis. In order to do this, physicians must consider chemical sensitivity when presented with a patient experiencing multi-system symptoms. Application of the differential diagnostic method will fail if the diagnosis is not considered. In addition to putting chemical sensitivity on the "to-rule-out" list, physicians must take a detailed exposure history, with focus on temporal associations between chemical

exposures and onset and/or worsening of symptoms. As attested to by
Dr. William Meggs in the Introduction to *Amputated Lives*, funds for
research in this area are basically nonexistent. As a result, pathophysiologic mechanisms are poorly understood and specific diagnostic
tests unavailable. Consequently the process of exclusion becomes more
important.

The second challenge for the physician is to treat his or her patient
appropriately. Simple recognition of the disease by a physician is an
important first step in treating the patient with chemical sensitivity. It
provides validation and an antidote to the all-too-common attribution of
symptoms to psychological problems. Beyond diagnosis of the disease,
effective treatment entails a thorough understanding by both physician
and patient of the minute details of the patient's environment. Because
environments change, the need for a careful exposure history and advice
on how to eliminate harmful exposures is ongoing. An example is
provided by Johnson in the case of Randa, who developed multiple
chemical sensitivity from chemical exposures associated with the installation of new carpeting in her office. She subsequently developed
reactions to the gas heat and gas stove in her apartment, and then to
mold. The latter prompted a move to New Mexico where the air is dry.
Unfortunately, the flat adobe roofs in that area often become leaky after
a few years, contributing to mold growth in spite of the generally dry
air. Randa was finally forced out of her apartment by exposures associated with the installation of new carpeting in the apartment of an
upstairs neighbor. Physicians can play a valuable role in providing
moral support and advice under such circumstances, offering common-
sense solutions that may not occur to the patient who is ill and likely
feeling overwhelmed.

For us as a society, the challenge is to prevent a preventable disease
that has become a public health problem. In Massachusetts, each year
the Governor recognizes multiple chemical sensitivity and its impact on
residents of the Commonwealth with the declaration of "Multiple
Chemical Sensitivity Awareness Week." But such tacit recognition is
not enough. We need acknowledgment and acceptance of chemical
sensitivity by the scientific community. We need funding for research
to identify the underlying pathophysiologic mechanisms of chemical
sensitivity and to develop effective treatment modalities. We need
funding for education of the U.S. population generally and health pro-

fessionals specifically with regard to chemical sensitivity. We need involvement of those who can make practical differences in the lives of those with the disease, including architects, building contractors, and manufacturers of chemical products used in home and building construction.

Amputated Lives aptly describes five situations in the recent history of our country in which action, if taken, could have prevented the occurrence of thousands of cases of chemical sensitivity: the laying of new carpet in the poorly ventilated EPA building in Washington, D.C., in 1987; the *Exxon Valdez* oil spill in 1989; the Gulf War in 1991; the terrorist attacks in 2001; and Hurricane Katrina in 2005. There will be more natural disasters, and there may be more wars and terrorist attacks. But our response does not have to be the same. Alison Johnson has issued a wake-up call with her book. Let's all listen.

L. Christine Oliver, MD, MPH, MS

Harvard Medical School

Preface

All my books and documentaries have had a central goal in mind–to convince readers and viewers that chemical sensitivity is real and is devastating far too many lives. In the ten years that have passed since I produced and directed my first documentary, *Multiple Chemical Sensitivity: How Chemical Exposures May Be Affecting Your Health*, more and more people have been succumbing to this condition. Hardly a day goes by that I do not hear from someone who is close to despair because they see their former life slipping away from them as they struggle with a condition that the medical profession has largely ignored.

Last month a taxicab driver from Las Vegas e-mailed to say: "I was making good money driving a taxi and had to resign because the other driver would spray it with air freshener. Eventually the cab made me so sick I had to quit." A man in a state prison wrote to say that he was getting terrible headaches from the scented products that his cell mate uses. Another e-mail came from a New York City police detective who toiled for months on the World Trade Center cleanup and is now too sick to work. He has become extremely sensitive to cleaning products, fragrances, and diesel exhaust and summed up his condition by saying, "I am beyond miserable."

An artist who has found it enormously difficult to find a place to live that she can tolerate expressed her frustration by writing: "In the search for a new home, I came to know full well an overwhelming feeling of desperation, and along with that desperation came the growing conviction that the chemically sensitive are viewed as 'throw away' people."

In Part II, people who are chemically sensitive describe in their own words how this has changed their lives forever. I have also used extensive quotes from these individuals in Part I instead of filtering their experience through my own words. It is my hope that this book will persuade readers that those unfortunate enough to have developed multiple chemical sensitivity are not "throw away" people, but the proverbial canaries in the mine alerting us that the rapid proliferation in chemical products in our environment may be endangering all of us.

Books by Alison Johnson

Casualties of Progress:
Personal Histories from the
Chemically Sensitive

Gulf War Syndrome:
Legacy of a Perfect War

**Documentaries Produced and
Directed by Alison Johnson**

Multiple Chemical Sensitivity:
How Chemical Exposures May
Be Affecting Your Health

Gulf War Syndrome:
Aftermath of a Toxic Battlefield

The Toxic Clouds of 9/11:
A Looming Health Disaster

www.alisonjohnsonmcs.com

About the Author

Alison Johnson, BA., M.A., is a summa cum laude graduate of Carleton College and studied mathematics at the Sorbonne on a National Science Foundation Fellowship. She received a master's degree in mathematics from the University of Wisconsin, where she studied on a Woodrow Wilson Fellowship. She developed chemical sensitivity at age thirty-five and became an advocate for the chemically sensitive after all three of her daughters developed the condition in their early teenage years. Unlike so many people with this condition, Johnson and her daughters are lucky enough to have their chemical sensitivity reasonably well under control through the avoidance of major chemical exposures.

Johnson has shown her films on Capitol Hill, at HUD and the EPA in Washington, D.C., and in London, Wiesbaden, Montreal, Ottawa, and Halifax, as well as in many U.S. cities. In February 2001, on the occasion of the tenth anniversary of the end of the Gulf War, she organized a press conference on Capitol Hill in which several veterans read excerpts from their stories in her book on Gulf War syndrome and Ross Perot and Senators Kay Bailey Hutchison and Dick Durbin spoke. Johnson's book *Casualties of Progress* will be appearing in Italian in 2009. All her works with the exception of her MCS documentary have been given to every member of Congress. Johnson chairs the Chemical Sensitivity Foundation, which she founded in 2001. In 2004, the American Academy of Environmental Medicine gave her its Carleton Lee Award for "exemplary efforts in furthering the principles of Environmental Medicine."

Acknowledgments

I wish to express my appreciation to several people who read extensive portions of the manuscript: Betsey Grobe, Joan Smith, Sue Renaud, and Bob Weggel. My thanks also go to my cousin Elizabeth Musick, who has once again designed a beautiful cover for me.

Part I

Introduction

Four cataclysmic events have rocked the United States in the last two decades: the 1989 *Exxon Valdez* oil spill, the 1991 Gulf War, the destruction of the World Trade Center in 2001, and Hurricane Katrina in 2005. At first glance, these events might seem to have little in common, but all left in their wake significant numbers of people who are now chronically ill after exposure to large amounts of toxic chemicals. Some were volunteers or held jobs that left them little choice; some were just in the wrong place at a very wrong time. Hundreds of thousands of Americans became the "designated fall-guys," finding themselves on the front lines of wars or natural disasters. During the cleanup operations in Alaska, at Ground Zero, and in the New Orleans area, thousands of people stepped forward to remove toxic substances in an effort to enable the pristine waters of Prince William Sound, the world's financial hub in Lower Manhattan, and the jazz capital of America to return to at least some semblance of normalcy.

Regrettably, the national attention span is short. The sick workers who helped clean up the oil from the Alaskan beaches are not on anyone's radar screen. Two whom I interviewed were coughing so hard because of the asthma they had developed after cleaning the beaches that we could hardly continue the conversation. In November 2000, the *American Journal of Epidemiology* published a study showing that 34 percent of those who served in the Gulf War–over 200,000 veterans–are now chronically ill.[1] The young men and women who answered their country's call to serve on what has been termed the most toxic battlefield in history have felt abandoned for over seventeen years.

Then there are the heroes who responded to the World Trade Center disaster. Slogans on bumper stickers and in store windows throughout New York proclaimed that the 9/11 heroes would never be forgotten. Now most feel they have indeed been forgotten as their health

---

[1] Lea Steele, "Prevalence and Patterns of Gulf War Illness in Kansas Veterans: Association of Symptoms with Characteristics of Person, Place, and Time of Military Service," *American Journal of Epidemiology* 152, no. 10 (2000): 993.

deteriorates and they lose their jobs and the medical insurance that went with those jobs. In the case of Katrina, neglect has been even more evident, and little has been done to acknowledge the widespread exposure to toxic chemicals and mold encountered by residents and cleanup workers.

Large numbers of people who became chronically ill after these major exposure events have developed a new sensitivity to the chemicals they encounter in everyday life in substances like perfume, paint, gasoline, cigarette smoke, diesel exhaust, new carpet, cleaning products, and air fresheners.

But before these four cataclysmic events, there was a minor prelude in 1987 that barely caused a ripple in the national attention. It was an event that, had its importance been realized, would have laid the groundwork for saving tens of thousands of people from developing chemical sensitivity as a result of the *Exxon Valdez* cleanup, the Gulf War, the terrorist attack on the World Trade Center, and Katrina.

What was this preliminary event? In 1987 the EPA installed thousands of square yards of what turned out to be particularly dubious new carpet in its Washington, D.C., headquarters, a building that had very poor ventilation. This new carpet sickened a large number of the lawyers, scientists, and others working in the building. Within a few months, the agency found itself faced with a dilemma that might not have seemed significant at the time but would have immense and far-reaching consequences for the health of not only affected EPA employees but other Americans from all walks of life–beauticians, teachers, custodians, nurses, mechanics, artists, Gulf War veterans, 9/11 First Responders–the list goes on and on. In the latter decades of the twentieth century, more and more people began to develop a newfound sensitivity to everyday chemicals, a condition that is now most commonly called "multiple chemical sensitivity," or MCS. This condition was first described in the 1950s by a visionary professor of allergy at Northwestern School of Medicine named Theron Randolph. Dr. Randolph soon lost his position for promoting the heretical idea that some people develop serious symptoms in response to low levels of chemical exposure.

The EPA's dilemma was this: should it carry out serious health evaluations to discover if its recent carpet installation had led to the development of chemical sensitivity among many of its employees or should it stonewall the situation, acting as if nothing was really wrong, and thereby avoid incurring the wrath of the carpet industry?

Unfortunately, the EPA chose to placate the carpet manufacturers and ignore its sick employees. Thus in 1987 the agency established to protect Americans from toxic substances in their environment failed to protect even the employees in its own national headquarters and thereby missed an opportunity to alert the nation to the insidious and potentially devastating condition of multiple chemical sensitivity (MCS). With classic cases developing within its own huge Washington office building, the agency was in an ideal position to study the phenomenon of MCS and encourage other high government agencies like the National Institutes of Health to devote substantial funds to research the condition.

If the EPA had alerted the nation to chemical sensitivity when it developed in its own headquarters in 1987, Exxon executives and the government officials who advised them would have been far less cavalier about letting hapless workers clean the oil-soaked beaches in Alaska while wearing minimal protective gear. And if the EPA had understood the tremendous effects that multiple chemical sensitivity can have on people's health, the agency might have thought twice about encouraging Exxon to spread on the oily beaches a coating of Inipol or Corexit, strong chemicals that were supposed to help break down the oil. Unfortunately, these products added to the workers' exposure to toxic substances, thereby increasing the possibility that large numbers of them would become sensitized to many other chemicals.

Had the EPA recognized the development of multiple chemical sensitivity in its own employees in 1987, the leaders of the medical profession and physicians across the country might have begun to take MCS seriously. They would then have been in a better position to recognize why so many veterans of the 1991 Gulf War were seeking medical help for a wide variety of chronic symptoms like headaches, asthma, joint and muscle pains, gastrointestinal problems, and severe memory loss. These veterans suffered for years in an increasing state of frustration while their health and financial situations were declining as the Department of Defense and the VA attributed their symptoms to stress.

Change comes very slowly in huge government bureaucracies, but Dr. Ronald Blanck, who was the U.S. Army Surgeon General and the Commander of Walter Reed Army Medical Center during much of the

1990s, was one leader who began to question the stress theory that assumed that the illnesses suffered by so many returning veterans were psychologically based. In my documentary *Gulf War Syndrome: Aftermath of a Toxic Battlefield*, 2004 version, Dr. Blanck states:

> In the mid-1990s, I commanded Walter Reed Army Medical Center. I continued to work on looking for causes for the illnesses suffered by many Gulf War veterans, illnesses that were clearly more than stress related. I looked at vaccines, I looked at exposure to smokes, to other toxic chemicals, petrochemicals, and so forth, all that were part of that battlefield experience, and I came to the conclusion that at least one of the explanations was multiple chemical sensitivity, something where a variety of toxic elements, even at low levels by themselves, in combination may in susceptible individuals be causing these illnesses. And I believe so much more work needs to be done on that, but it is clearly one of the explanations.
>
> Although there's been increased recognition that there are causes other than stress for these illnesses, really the sea change happened in the last year or so and is highlighted by an article in the *New York Times* of October 15, 2004, that states many of the ill veterans "suffer from neurologic damage caused by exposure to toxic chemicals."

A decade separated the Gulf War from 9/11, but the EPA learned nothing during this period. Instead, the political appointees heading the EPA circled the wagons in response to a lawsuit initiated in 1992 by a group of its sick employees, who claimed that exposure to new carpet fumes and other renovation substances had caused them to develop multiple chemical sensitivity. As a result, when the planes struck the World Trade Center towers, MCS was not high on the list of potential health risks at Ground Zero for Christine Todd Whitman, the head of the national EPA, or for the official who headed the EPA office in New York City. These EPA officials did nothing to warn the tens of thousands of people who toiled in the toxic clouds at Ground Zero to help clean up the World Trade Center debris or those who lived and worked in the area blanketed by smoke for weeks that among other risks to their health, the development of MCS would be a very troubling possibility. None of these people were warned that MCS would have the potential to change their lives forever, eventually making it difficult for them to find a workplace or apartment or house they could tolerate, as is sadly illustrated by Chapters One and Two.

In a 1999 article in *Archives of Environmental Health* that was titled "Multiple Chemical Sensitivity: A 1999 Consensus," a group of thirty-four researchers and clinicians proposed the following criteria for the clinical diagnosis of MCS:

1. The symptoms are reproducible with repeated exposure.
2. The condition is chronic.
3. Low levels of exposure result in manifestations of the syndrome.
4. The symptoms improve or resolve when the incitants are removed.
5. Responses occur to multiple chemically unrelated substances.
6. Symptoms involve multiple organ systems.

One of the most distinctive features of MCS is that people who develop the condition begin to react to low-level chemical exposures that never bothered them previously. Some MCS patients have only mild cases; for others the condition can be life threatening. In most cases, as the illness progresses, the patient reports that more and more substances cause symptoms. People with MCS can have a wide variety of symptoms as the result of chemical exposures, with different patients having different symptoms. A given patient, however, will usually have the same symptom in response to a given exposure, perhaps getting a headache after exposure to paint or getting arthritic pains after exposure to natural gas.

Even though researchers do not yet agree on a precise definition for the condition, the stories in Part II illustrate how chemical sensitivity can destroy a productive life all too quickly. Many people with MCS are so sensitive to fragrances that they virtually become prisoners in their own home, unable to go to church, work, classes, or social gatherings because they will react to the perfume, aftershave, shampoos, detergents, or fabric softeners used by others. To make matters worse, some of those who insist that MCS is a psychologically based illness state that these people are suffering from agoraphobia, or fear of crowds. That's as cruel as saying to a paraplegic in a wheelchair, "Too bad you don't like to walk."

Newspaper reporters often refer to multiple chemical sensitivity as a rare condition, but this is hardly the case. In 2004, *Archives of Environmental Health* published a national prevalence study by Stanley Caress and Anne Steinemann.[2] These researchers reported that in their national random phone survey, 2.5 percent of the respondents said that they had been diagnosed with MCS. This result suggests that over seven million Americans may be suffering from multiple chemical sensitivity, a number that exceeds the population of Massachusetts. This is hardly a "rare condition," as it is frequently termed in the media.

The potential for MCS to gradually increase a person's sensitivity to the point that he or she can't find a workplace that can be tolerated leads to a situation in which large numbers of chemically sensitive people eventually end up with no choice but to turn to public assistance like SSSI (Social Security Supplemental Income). This is yet another reason why the medical profession and government bodies should turn their attention to a condition that has the potential to be a huge drain on public finances.

The loss to society of the contributions of teachers, mechanics, nurses, and others is significant. A case in point is a highly intelligent young woman who appears in my documentary *The Toxic Clouds of 9/11: A Looming Health Disaster;* her story appears in Part II of this book. Jenn Duncan received her B.S. degree from MIT and her M.S. degree from New York University. One of the jobs she loved most was working for the Children's Television Workshop, which produced "Sesame Street. " Ironically enough, when Jenn developed severe MCS and lost the ability to think clearly enough to read and write, she taught herself to read again by watching *Sesame Street*. One of the great regrets of her life is that she is no longer in a position to contribute to society by doing the creative work she loved so much.

By contrast, Victoria Savini, who has a less severe case of MCS than Jenn, has been able to keep working. She developed multiple chemical sensitivity while working in the accounts payable office of the Disburse-

---

[2] Stanley Caress and Anne Steinemann, "Prevalence of Hypersensitivity to Common Chemicals: A National Population Study," *Archives of Environmental Health*, 59, no. 6 (2004): 300-305.

ment Division of the Hart Senate Office Building. Because two letters containing anthrax spores were sent to senators in the Hart Building during the 2001 anthrax scare, the building was fumigated. In addition, in order to protect against contaminated mail, the government started irradiating all mail coming into congressional offices. This irradiation process had an extreme effect upon the paper, causing some of it to turn yellow and disintegrate on its edges, as I saw in person when I visited a congressional office during this period. I was also told that the young staffer who opened the bag of office mail every day felt nauseated by the fumes she inhaled. Victoria describes in her story in Part II how she had to leave her Senate job after she became chemically sensitive. Fortunately, she was able to find work with a major foundation in the Washington area that was willing to accommodate her MCS. As a result of this enlightened policy, Victoria has been able to work productively for the past seven years.

With MCS affecting millions of Americans, why is there so little recognition of the condition and why has so little money been spent to research it? In their book *Chemical Exposures: Low Levels and High Stakes,* Nicholas Ashford, Ph.D., J.D., and Claudia Miller, M.D., M.S., two of the leading authorities in the field, explore this issue. The *Journal of the American Medical Association* described their book as "a stimulating review of the controversy surrounding multiple chemical sensitivities" and also said, "Clinicians and policymakers would do well to read and heed the advice of this book." Ashford and Miller decry the lack of research funds for MCS:

> Scientific investigation related to chemical sensitivity is being stymied by scientists and physicians with financial conflicts of interest (e.g., those working for the chemical industry and those acting as defense expert witnesses in legal cases on MCS) who serve on government panels, editorial review boards, and grant review committees. These conflicts generally remain undisclosed.
>
> Ashford & Miller, p. 271

One of the most respected researchers in the field of chemical sensitivity is William Meggs, M.D., Ph.D., a toxicologist and professor at East Carolina University Brody School of Medicine. Dr. Meggs has published many articles in peer-reviewed journals detailing, among other topics, his research using biopsies to investigate damage to the nasal lining of chemically sensitive patients. When I interviewed Dr. Meggs for my documentary on MCS, he stated:

> I've spent a lot of time applying for research grants to try to study these illnesses and the role of chemicals in these illnesses, and my grant applications come back with scathing comments [like] "Don't spend any money on this research because everybody knows this is all psychological."

It's hardly surprising that industry doesn't want anyone to believe that chemical exposures could produce a debilitating condition like MCS. The consequences for corporations would be enormous if members of the public increasingly began to wonder if installing new carpet, using pesticides in their house or yard, or buying particleboard cabinets or furniture might affect their health. And imagine the potential liability problems if people could prove that exposures in factories, hospitals, schools, or offices had destroyed their health.

To understand the power that industry wields regarding MCS, one need only remember that the tobacco industry managed for decades to keep the public from recognizing the hazards of smoking. They were able to succeed in this agenda not only by funding research that would encourage people to think that smoking was safe, but also by discouraging any research that might show the dangers of smoking. If the tobacco industry, which represents a very small fraction of American business, could exercise so much power, it is indeed staggering to consider the influence against validating MCS that is wielded by corporations when almost every business in the United States is significantly involved in chemical use in one way or another. What advertiser would want to run ads on a TV show that raised the possibility that chemical exposures could be creating serious illness? Certainly not advertisers from the cosmetic, pesticide, construction, or carpet industries.

In their book, Ashford and Miller also discuss at length psychological issues related to MCS. They make the important point that while some MCS patients have psychiatric symptoms from time to time, that does not mean that the illness is psychological in origin. An illustrative example is Mad Hatter's disease from the nineteenth century; the Mad

Hatters were indeed crazy, but their insanity was caused by the mercury in the felt with which they worked. One study has shown that panic disorder can be precipitated by exposure to solvents in the workplace.[3]

A particularly telling argument against the theory that MCS is simply a psychological condition related to a fear of chemicals comes from animal research. Several recent experiments replicate features of MCS in a rodent animal model, showing that rodents can react with debilitating symptoms to extremely low levels of chemicals. These rodents are obviously not influenced by media accounts of the dangers of chemical exposure. This area of research clearly cries out for funding.

Another unfortunate aspect of the psychological approach to the issue of chemical sensitivity is that critics of MCS frequently suggest that "secondary gain" is a strong component of the condition. According to secondary gain theorists, those with MCS are engaging in certain behavior patterns in order to get special attention or because they want others to take care of them. One does not have to read many of the stories in Part II before it becomes apparent that this suggestion at best is made in ignorance and at worst represents an exceedingly cruel attitude toward people whose illness has in all too many cases cost them their job, their home, their friends, or their spouse. MCS is in all too many cases an illness of devastating and overwhelming loss, not secondary gain. John, a former Shakespeare professor living with chemical sensitivity, described his situation in these poignant words:

> I have been told that early retirement is the American dream. Early retirement because of disability and a chronic, progressive illness is nothing but a bad dream, involving the loss of family, home, career, friends, mobility, income, and one's health— almost everything one holds precious.
>
> *Casualties of Progress*, p. 162

Nor is "secondary gain" a phrase that would come to mind when one reads the words of Randa, a woman who had worked in a land-use planning office in California and enjoyed activities like hiking in the Himalayas before she developed MCS:

---

[3] Stephen Dager et al., "Panic Disorder Precipitated by Exposure to Organic Solvents in the Work Place," *American Journal of Psychiatry* 144, no. 8 (1987): 1056-58.

Living with chemical sensitivity is being chronically ill and feeling crummy most of the time. After nine years of that, it really wears on you. It's really tiring, and I don't know how to explain this condition to people. It's drudgery and monotonous and lonely and isolating, and your old friends and your family don't want to hear about it, and I don't want to hear about it, but it's my life.

Casualties of Progress, p. 138

The concept of secondary gain would also hardly apply to two chemically sensitive people who recently told me how MCS has affected them:

MCS has had a profound impact on my life. I went from a life of plans and dreams–like getting married and having a family–to a life of constant struggle. During my sixteen years of illness, there have been literally hundreds of days of frustration, isolation, and extreme discomfort. Every day becomes a challenge to minimize the exposures that will make me sick. But the exposures are everywhere and never-ending: scented fabric softener fumes from a neighbor's dryer vent, nearby pesticide spraying, a co-worker using perfume or cologne, toxic cleaners used on a store floor, and office buildings with out-gassing synthetic materials, etc. Surviving this burden for so many years has undoubtedly been the greatest accomplishment of my life–an amazing accomplishment that will go completely unnoticed by most of the people I know.

Eric

Getting MCS has meant that within a year I lost my job of $40,000 a year as a social worker, I lost my boyfriend of four years, and basically lost my home, as I could not sleep in it. Having MCS has meant enormous difficulties in finding work even if I have five degrees, including a Ph.D., as there are so many indoor environments I can't tolerate.

Nathalie

Reading *Amputated Lives* should quickly dispel any thought that people who suffer from chemical sensitivity are simply malingering. Far too many chemically sensitive people are living desperate lives, not lives spent in comfort while others care for them.

Chapter 1

The Struggle to Find
a Safe Workplace

Work is key to our existence. It pays the bills for us and our families. It helps define us as a person. But what happens when the ability to work becomes almost beyond reach because one reacts to chemical exposures in the workplace?

It's not easy to find a job where chemical exposures are not a problem. Fragrances are ubiquitous in almost all workplaces. Most factory jobs involve substantial exposures to toxic chemicals; health care facilities use heavy amounts of cleaning products and disinfectants, which are in effect dilute pesticides; and office air is polluted by the fumes from printers, copiers, and computers. And forget any kind of job that involves mechanical skills since exposure to diesel, gasoline, oil, and lubricants are out of the question for the chemically sensitive.

Jay Wilcoxen was very sensitive to chemicals after he came home from the 1991 Gulf War. When he retired from the military and took a job driving a truck, he would vomit every time he put diesel in his vehicle. During the Gulf War, Patricia Browning drove a tractor-trailer truck. Like so many other soldiers, she came home with Gulf War syndrome, with its accompanying chemical sensitivity, and this severely impacted her ability to drive a truck. In her story in my book *Casualties of Progress*, Pat writes, "I was a reservist for a number of years after the Gulf War, but even when I didn't need a cane anymore, I couldn't drive a truck because every time they would crank up the trucks, I would get deathly ill."

Randa had to give up her good job in a land-use planning office in California when she developed chemical sensitivity after a new carpet was glued down. When I filmed her in 1998 for my video on multiple chemical sensitivity, she said, "I haven't worked for over ten years now, and that really does a job on your self-esteem." Make that twenty years now that Randa has been unable to work.

Richard was a very successful painting contractor before his workplace exposures sensitized him to a wide variety of chemicals. Like

Randa, he found that being unable to work had a huge effect on his sense of his personal worth:

> I think especially as a man, not being able to work was very difficult. For all of my adult life, I guess I had identified with what I was doing for a job and had identified with my role as a business owner, someone who was providing employment for other people, someone who was performing a service for people, someone who got a big fat paycheck when the job was done.
>
> *Casualties of Progress*, p. 115

Michael owned a large tree and pesticide business in which he sprayed over 100,000 gallons of pesticide every year. When he eventually developed MCS, he found it especially difficult when he was unable to work:

> People—my wife, my family, other people, my brother especially—used to complain about what a workaholic I was, how I was just unbelievably driven, I would never stop. I would work weekends, I would work till dark. I just couldn't get enough. Going from being a workaholic to wondering how you're going to provide for your wife and your two children is pretty tough to take, especially as a male in this society. Society expects you to provide for your family, and people look at you strangely when you don't seem to be working your normal forty hours or more.
>
> *Casualties of Progress*, p. 11

National Guard Captain Richard Caron developed Gulf War syndrome and chemical sensitivity after his service in Desert Storm. In his case the severe memory loss this condition often causes made it almost impossible for him to work, as he recounts:

> Before I went to the Gulf War, I had a full-time job as a carpenter. I was also the pastor of a Baptist church and the chaplain of my Army National Guard unit. . . .
>
> I have had to make many adjustments in my life because of the chemical sensitivity I had brought back from the Gulf War. I had to give up my job as pastor at my church because I was having a hard time remembering scripture passages that I used to know by heart.

Because the construction trade was slow at the time I returned from the war, I got a job in law enforcement because I had previous experience in the field. I worked for the sheriff's department for a while and also for a city police department. I wasn't able to continue that line of work, however, because I had become very forgetful since my return from the war and would get confused about where I was. There would be times when I'd be out driving on roads that I'd traveled many times before, and sometimes I couldn't remember where I was. I would just have to keep going, and finally I would realize where I was. When I was trying to work in law enforcement, I would get a call to go to a certain location where something was happening, and I couldn't remember where that street was located. So I just had to give up that work.

Casualties of Progress, pp. 62-63

Sgt. James Green is a young man who developed multiple chemical sensitivity while he was in the Air Force:

My memory is so bad now that I can't even drive on back roads here where I've driven since I was sixteen because I forget which way to go. I also became very sensitive to various chemicals; I can't stand being around cleaning chemicals, and diesel fumes or exhaust always gave me horrible headaches. Finally I just couldn't keep working around all the diesel exposures on the flight line, so I left the Air Force. For a couple of months, I drove a truck for a man who was laying cable for TV's, and the only way that worked was that he told me where to go and when to turn. The worst thing was that my diarrhea was so bad that we would have to stop every half hour for me to use a bathroom. Of course, after a while I had to quit that job.

Casualties of Progress, p. 99

One particularly poignant description of a long struggle to find a job he could tolerate comes from Abner Fisch, who worked productively as a chemical engineer for a dozen years before he developed MCS. At a 1996 hearing held by the Governor's Committee on the Needs of the Handicapped in Santa Fe, New Mexico, Abner testified about the problems he had encountered in his search for a job:

I've had MCS since 1984. Since 1984, I've had twenty different employments. I've been looking very hard for steady employment, and it seems to be elusive. Two things are very difficult for people with MCS. One is that there are many jobs we just cannot do because of new carpet or carbonless carbon paper or new equipment or employees wearing perfume. Another problem for people with MCS is that when we have a job, sometimes we have to resign our job because of changes in the environment that take place.

I graduated as a chemical engineer in 1971. I worked for five years for two different state governments in pollution control, and then I started to work for 3M. . . . When I acquired MCS in 1984, 3M tried to accommodate me. They transferred me from a chemical pilot plant to an office job, but at that particular time, I was too sensitive to function well and I received a very bad performance evaluation. . . .

I had several jobs, and I went back to school and got a teaching certificate in Minnesota, and I have done substitute teaching there.

I've applied for many jobs. I applied for a job with the city of St. Paul which would require me to work with carbonless carbon paper. After the interview, I told them I couldn't do the job. Shortly after I left 3M, I applied for a job as a consulting engineer, but I couldn't wear the clothes, nor could I work in the building with new carpet.

Just last week I applied for a job in the Questa elementary schools, and the superintendent, Señor Gonzales, . . . took me into the building. Within a couple of minutes, I knew that I would get dizzy and disorganized and I would be irritable with the children. I couldn't justify being a teacher and being irritable with the children because of the physical structure of the building. It's just not fair to kids. So I told Señor Gonzales I couldn't do it.

In other cases, there have been jobs I had to quit because new carpet was installed. I had a job as a counselor in a halfway house and had to quit the job when carpeting was put in. I was a personal care attendant, and when the family remodeled the house and put in new carpet, I had to quit. I was flipping burgers and running a cash register, and I got a very good performance evaluation after two months and after four months, but when they hired new employees who wore perfume and kept scheduling me with them, I had to resign.

I do substitute teaching, and when I substitute teach, every day when I come home I have to wash my clothing to get the perfume off.

Casualties of Progress, pp. 144-45

Six months after he gave this testimony, Abner took his own life. Lynn Lawson, the former editor of the *Canary News*, the newsletter of the Chicago MCS group, told me that two or three weeks before he ended his life, Abner called her to ask if she knew of any housing anywhere in the country that would be safe for MCS people. His suicide was almost certainly related to the two major problems facing those with MCS: finding a safe place to work and finding a safe place to live.

As chair of the Chemical Sensitivity Foundation, I frequently receive e-mails from desperate people, and it's not easy to know what to reply. The following message came in February 2005:

I have been plagued with multiple chemical sensitivities for about fourteen years, ever since the carpets in my home were cleaned and treated with a stain-repellent chemical.

My biggest concern is finding an occupation and/or workplace for someone with my problems. I don't know if this is something that your organization can help me with, but I'm at my wit's end and don't know where to turn. I need and want to work; I have started and had to quit so many wonderful jobs in the past four years due to becoming sick in the workplace.

If you have any information on how a MCS person can obtain gainful employment, I would be deeply grateful.

What can society offer this woman? She wants a job, not a handout. Some way must be found to accommodate such people in at least some workplaces so that they can remain productive members of society. Given the rather alarming increase in MCS during the last decade, there is some potential for the number of people needing public assistance to overwhelm the Social Security Disability Income and Supplemental Income programs if this growing problem is not addressed.

Chapter 2

The Elusive Search for
a Place to Live

Chemically sensitive people face a difficult struggle to find a place to live that will not exacerbate their health problems, a struggle that sometimes can seem almost overwhelming. Some people who are chemically sensitive are so reactive to the carpet or paint or gas heat in their living quarters or to their neighbors' use of pesticides or dryer sheets that they end up feeling lousy on bad days and half-sick most of the rest of the time. An exposure that might seem slight to the ordinary person can cause the intense pain and nausea of a migraine that can last for a couple of days or it can bring on an asthma attack. In other cases, an exposure can produce a dull headache or joint or muscle pains that make it hard for people to accomplish what they would like to do. Some exposures leave susceptible people feeling exhausted for days.

The chemically sensitive are often driven to lengths that to others seem astonishing, if not downright unbelievable, as various excerpts from the personal histories in my book *Casualties of Progress* illustrate. A former college English professor named John reports that his chemical sensitivity originated when he was exposed to pesticide fogging while attending graduate school in Gainesville, Florida. Despite various resulting health problems, he was able to teach in the State University of New York system for ten years. Then in 1978 when his college remodeled the building in which he taught, putting in new carpet, painting the walls with an oil-based paint, and introducing a new floor wax, twenty-six teachers became so sick that they signed a petition protesting their working conditions. The floor wax, which contained a formaldehyde preservative, was withdrawn from the market the following year. Unfortunately, these new exposures to toxic chemicals caused John such health problems that he had to give up his career as a college professor. Like many others with chemical sensitivity, he eventually moved to the desert Southwest, where his extreme sensitivity to building materials caused him to adopt a highly unusual lifestyle:

I once read a study that said the average American spends 98% of the day inside. I've reversed that proportion and spend 98% of my time outdoors, sleeping on my patio and cooking there on a hot plate. I use my house as an oversized closet, storage area, and bathroom. I've been basically living outdoors for twenty years now.

Casualties of Progress, p. 161

Michael owned a very successful pesticide company in Connecticut and supervised the spraying of 100,000 gallons of pesticide every year. Not surprisingly, he developed chemical sensitivity after a few years of this exposure. When Michael's chemical sensitivity forced him to sell his large pesticide business, he moved to a farm in northern New England. His wife Judy describes in *Casualties of Progress* the problems they experienced while trying to make the farmhouse they had bought livable:

After we renovated our farmhouse with all nontoxic substances, we moved in in a flurry pace. Within 48 hours, however, Michael was sleeping outside on the porch under five wool blankets and three sleeping bags because he was unable to live in the house. It was November, and it was beginning to snow, so he was really freezing out there. We had been renovating the house for four months, and Michael had been in the house every single day with no problem until the last two or three weeks when we were working on the kitchen floor. We were having it laid with linoleum flooring, and Michael noticed he was losing his voice and not feeling very good. We are convinced that the glue that was holding the linoleum to the floor was what pushed Michael out the door. He was unable to enter the house for another month after that except for very short periods of time. When he did, you could see a red rash develop on his face and he would get beady eyes, glassy, watery eyes.

Casualties of Progress, p. 15

After Randa developed extreme chemical sensitivity because of new carpeting glued down in her office, she started reacting to her gas heat and gas stove. She had to turn off the gas and buy electric heaters, an electric toaster oven, and a hot plate. Mold had never bothered her in the past, but now she started to react to it, so she had to rip out her carpeting, which was slightly moldy. She followed her doctor's suggestion and moved to Santa Fe because of her new and troublesome mold sensitivity, but that did not solve the problem:

> My particular problem in finding housing here in Santa Fe is that the majority of houses are pueblo-style architecture and have flat roofs that typically leak when the houses are over ten years old. The leaks cause irreparable mold in the roofs. If I walk into a house that is over ten years old, it's almost always too moldy for me and my lungs tighten up immediately.
>
> *Casualties of Progress*, p. 139

After looking at about two hundred places in Santa Fe, Randa found a condo that worked fairly well for a while until new carpet in an adjacent apartment caused her serious problems:

> Unfortunately, my upstairs neighbor installed new carpet at the beginning of summer, and that made me homeless for over three months until the carpet had outgassed enough that it was tolerable for me. As soon as the carpet was installed, my apartment filled with toxic chemicals and made me very ill and I had to leave right away. I had to sleep on friends' porches for many weeks.
>
> *Casualties of Progress*, p. 140

Randa did not consider building her own house to be a good option:

> I really haven't thought seriously about building my own house because many people with MCS who have built their own houses have had disasters and have not been able to move into their places for a long time (sometimes years). I am so exquisitely sensitive to building materials that it would be very hard for me to build a house that I could move into immediately. At least with an existing house, I can walk in and get an idea whether it will work. . . . The financial risk is just too great if it doesn't work.
>
> *Casualties of Progress,* p. 139

A graphic artist named Ariel had very mixed success with various attempts to find safe housing. Her odyssey started after she developed chemical sensitivity that she attributes to a computer printer at work that was improperly vented. As her health grew worse, she and her husband decided to take early retirement and move out of the city to a rural area on the western slope of the Colorado Rockies. Unfortunately, it didn't occur to them that living right next to an orchard was not a good idea. Ariel later described this experience:

> Each time the farmer sprayed his trees, I reacted with symptoms that were frighteningly severe—face and hand numbness, a total inability to focus my eyes, an extreme pressure in my head . . . chills that seemed to turn the marrow of my bones to ice and produced uncontrollable shivering. . . . These initial symptoms would gradually give way to a chronic flu-like state that involved bone-wracking aches, extreme fatigue, and difficulty breathing.
> . . . . . .
> Because the severity of the reactions I suffered with each spray event indicated that future exposures could result in anaphylactic shock, my doctor recommended that we move to an area free of pesticides. So in 1991 we moved to a beautiful valley where we felt safe behind the twenty miles we knew separated us from the nearest agricultural areas, where there might be herbicide or pesticide spraying.
> We bought a house and made the necessary changes to create a nontoxic home, adding a large artist studio for my work. We planted extensive gardens of vegetables, fruits, and berries to assure a pesticide-free food source.
> . . . . . .
> In 1997 my illusion of safety fell apart when an extensive noxious weed containment program was instituted in our area. . . . In the search for a new home, I came to know full well an overwhelming feeling of desperation, and along with that desperation came the growing conviction that the chemically sensitive are viewed as "throw away" people.
>
> *Casualties of Progress*, pp. 121-22

Ariel and her husband finally located a house they thought she could tolerate, only to find that the previous owners' assurances that they had used no pesticides in the house were incorrect. In the crawl space, they discovered several insecticide bombs whose lot numbers indicated they had been used by the previous owners. Faced with an extremely difficult choice, Ariel and her husband decided to build a new house on the property. They slept all winter in their trailer and camper, using the bathroom and laundry facilities in the original house while they built their new one. It was not an easy decision, as Ariel recounted:

> The necessity to build a new house has required us to cash in the last of our IRA's and other savings accounts. . . . . It's taken a large amount of mental fortitude and energy to pick up and start all over, to trust that we'll get it right this time and will not have to move again. We have once again cleared the brush, put up a deer fence, tilled and planted a large garden, planted fruit trees and berries. . . . Once again we are facing the dilemma that so many MCS people and their families face: spending down their income and savings to accommodate their illness, with no guarantees, no protective laws, no safety nets, and little basis for hope.
>
> *Casualties of Progress*, p. 123

A woman named Marian had developed such serious health problems related to her chemical sensitivity that she decided to move to the middle of the desert in southwestern New Mexico. For the first year or two she was there, her husband had to continue working elsewhere, although he eventually retired and joined her in the middle of the desert. In her story that she sent me in 1998, Marian described in poignant and haunting terms how difficult it had been to leave her old life and house behind and the challenges she had faced in moving to an isolated desert home. Unfortunately, she died in 2003.

> I was very ill. We took the recommendation to avoid toxic chemicals to heart. We sold our comfortable bed, the couch that I had selected with so much care, the chairs that complemented it. . . . The recliners we had relaxed in for years were given away. Sewing, knitting, crochet projects were thrown out half finished. Much of our clothing went with them. The carpets were torn up,

the gas pipes disconnected. Books, housewares, personal belongings, little things of no value and little things of great value, important parts of our lives were discarded with abandon in our zeal to clean up our house and improve our health.

An attractive and comfortable house in a pleasant setting is very important to me. I cannot easily shut out my surroundings. I get nourishment and comfort from what is around me. My body is gradually recovering as the toxic level that surrounds it has decreased, but the emotional cost of making the changes was enormous. The psychological effect of seeing the house I had so carefully furnished and decorated and made into a comfortable house turned into a bare and ugly barn was devastating, especially at a time when I was physically very, very debilitated and much in need of a comfortable and supportive environment.

. . . . .

I get lonely living by myself in the middle of the desert, so one day on a whim I tucked some snapshots around the light switch over my desk: My husband having breakfast outdoors wearing the slouchy hat I made for him, a bunch of wildflowers on the table in front of him. My older son, smiling at the camera as he squats beside a huge agave plant. My younger son, a tiny figure perched on top of an enormous rock, spreading his arms wide to soak up the warmth and beauty of the world. My daughter in a moment of attentive repose, looking up to watch her children at play.

Some days I talk to myself. I could talk to my husband, but he is presently living and working more than 200 miles away. I could visit our neighbors, but their home is full of chemicals. I could call a friend on the phone, but the phone is plastic. I could go hiking with some of the Mountain Club members, but they all use scented products. I could get together with a friend who also has chemical sensitivities, but the closest one is sixty miles away and that is a long drive in a smelly car on a smelly highway. I could talk to my dog and two cats (and sometimes do), but they don't answer, at least, not in words. But there are times when it gets too lonely if I don't hear the sound of a live human voice, so some days I talk to myself.

I try not to dwell on how seldom I see my family, how seldom I get to hug them, to share a meal with them, to enjoy the feel of their company. I try not to notice how my grandchildren are growing up without my getting to know them very well, or their getting to know me and my husband very well. I try not to realize the great physical distance and separation my chemical sensitivities have put between me and my family. I try very hard not to think of these things, for there is a great empty, aching void inside me when I do.

One of the strongest motivating forces in helping me endure my present life of isolating avoidance is the hope, the dream, the expectation that some day my children and grandchildren and my husband and I can move more freely between our two worlds.

Carina was an executive secretary for a large railroad who started to become chemically sensitive after she moved into a brand new apartment that contained particleboard cupboards, new carpets, and a gas furnace in a closet. She eventually bought a condo and made the mistake of pesticiding it because she thought previous owners might have had pets.

[I started] reacting to many different chemicals and had to flee my pesticide-contaminated condo and leave all my clothing and furniture behind me. I moved into a stripped-down apartment with no furniture and slept on a pallet on the floor. During this period, I was living on savings and waiting and worrying every day whether my application for disability would be approved. Thank God, it was. I was able to find someone to rent my condo, furnished, until I sold it. The loss of my belongings wasn't hard to take in the beginning, as I learned you could live without "things" in your life. But now, I seem to feel the loss more because I identified with all my things.

I found housing with an MCS couple [in Nevada] and stayed there almost three years. But when the couple got a divorce, I lost my safe housing and could find no other place to live. I went back to Arizona, where I spent almost a year moving from one temporary place to another. Many times I slept in my car. I couldn't handle this nomadic life physically, emotionally, or financially, however, so I returned to polluted southeastern Michigan, where my aunt took me in. I've been in her not-very-safe house for eight years now.

Casualties of Progress, pp. 150-51

Joy, whose chemical sensitivity would appear to be the result of her former work as a beautician and exposure to pesticides when their Arizona house was treated for termites, was forced to seek a new house. She hasn't succeeded in finding a safe place to live, as she explains:

We were in such a hurry to move so that I would feel better that we bought a home we knew we should never have moved into. We called the builder, and he told us their homes had very little particleboard; it was just used in the floor. The former owners swore they had never sprayed and never used scented products. They were such "nice" people that I believed them. But it turned out that I couldn't go in the house after the first time I tried because I got so dizzy. Thinking it was the thick new carpet making me sick, we had a subfloor put in and $9,000 worth of tile before we moved in. . . .

We stayed a month in a motel trying to heat and air out the house. Finally as funds were about to give out, we moved in and found that the cabinets that looked like hardwood were hardwood only on the doors. Every drawer, closet, and cabinet was made of particleboard, even the material under the counters.

The closets had been sprayed with pesticide, so I have to keep my clothes on racks in the bathroom because I cannot even open the door to the huge walk-in closet. The washer and dryer that came with the house took months to air out because the previous owners had used scented detergents and fabric softeners. I cannot open the doors to the cabinets where the detergents were kept.

We thought that because the area was desert and no lawns, there would be no pesticide spraying. Wrong! The neighbors spray every weed that grows so it will be nice sandy landscaping. I cannot open my windows in the summer. The neighbors also burn wood, and the smoke comes right into our house when the wind is in our direction.

We immediately put the house up for sale because of the formaldehyde gassing out of the particleboard, . . . but after trying to find a safer place for me to live, we finally took the house off the market. We did this in fear that another place might be worse than this one. We came to this decision after looking for a safe place and finding none. At our age we are just too tired to try again. I am seventy and my husband is seventy-three.

So each day I live in fear of my neighbors using their herbicides and pesticides, as I am bedridden for two to three weeks each time they do.

Casualties of Progress, pp. 208-9

Neighbors' use of pesticide led indirectly to the death of Nancy Noren, a computer systems analyst who was extremely sensitive to pesticides. According to an October 3, 1998, article in the *Albuquerque Tribune*:

A life-threatening disease often forced Nancy Noren to flee her Rio Rancho home in the middle of the night to find refuge and a few hours' sleep on a remote mesa. But it was on that mesa that the 51-year-old Rio Rancho woman may have met her death. Authorities confirmed Friday that a partly concealed body found earlier this week west of Albuquerque was Noren, who had been reported missing since July 17.

The police eventually arrested a twenty-two-year-old man who was stopped for speeding while he was driving Nancy's truck. Notes he had written indicated that he had been stalking Nancy on the mesa for some time. He was tried and convicted for her murder.

Friends of Nancy relate how her extreme sensitivity to the pesticides that her neighbors sprayed on their lawns affected her. One friend reported:

Nancy was totally incapacitated by pesticides and told me that it affected her whole body. The worst thing was that some of her neighbors were just not willing to talk about it at all and were quite rude about it. She wanted to ask them if they would at least warn her before applying pesticides so she could have the windows and doors closed, but they weren't even willing to do that.

When she would detect that pesticide had been sprayed, she would fly around the house closing windows as fast as possible, but it would still get in and cause her lots of pain. That's why on bad days she would have to just abandon the house and go walk on the mesa for most of the day. When the pesticide fumes were really bad, she would take her truck and camp in the camper shell on the back for a few days. Most of the time she camped out on the mesa because in a campground the charcoal lighter fluid and the cleaning products in the restrooms were a major problem for her.

Casualties of Progress, pp. 156-57

One of Nancy's other friends wrote:

Nancy realized her home was no longer good for her to be in, but she really couldn't conceive of moving for both financial and physical reasons, and we all know how difficult it is for people with MCS to find safe, affordable housing. She admitted to being overwhelmed by the idea of having to move.

Casualties of Progress, p. 157

Many people with MCS have committed suicide because they were unable to find housing that did not make them terribly sick. As the personal histories in my book *Casualties of Progress* illustrate all too well, many others across the country are living desperate lives. Some may be about to give up. Nancy Noren would be alive today had she been able to find suitable housing where she wasn't exposed to pesticides.

Finding safe housing is crucial for an individual attempting to climb out of the mire of MCS because living with constant exposure to toxic chemicals usually exacerbates or perpetuates the condition. Three national studies have shown that avoidance of chemical exposures is about the only therapy that seems to help virtually everyone with MCS feel better and regain some degree of health.[1] In some cases, a period of avoidance allows people with MCS the opportunity to reduce their level of sensitivity to chemicals sufficiently to enable them to work once again and to move about more freely in society.

The issue of constructing housing developments that could be viable for the chemically sensitive is not an easy one to handle because people with MCS do not all tolerate the same building materials. A useful first step, however, would be for some public-spirited developers to create developments that would reduce toxic exposures in the outside air. Such developments would benefit not only those with multiple chemical sensitivity but also those with asthma and other respiratory diseases. In such communities, it would be important to have bans on wood stoves or fireplaces, pesticides, smoking, barbecues, and the use of fabric softeners or dryer sheets, which spread fumes through a wide area surrounding the dryer vent. If the outdoor environment were protected in this way, then individuals could build their own houses using materials that they think they can tolerate and be free to open their windows to get some fresh air.

The need for such housing developments is immense. They would be a lifeline for people like the woman who sent me this e-mail in December 2005:

> I have Multiple Chemical Sensitivities so severe that I have had to resort to living in my vehicle in a National Forest in _____ for the past 14 months. I suffer severe neurological disturbances with exposures. Over the years my brain function has greatly diminished & I have become less able to fight the seemingly fruitless battle for housing & proper medical documentation. I

---

[1]Pamela Gibson et al., "Perceived Treatment Efficacy for Conventional and Alternative Therapies Reported by Persons with Multiple Chemical Sensitivity,"*Environmental Health Perspectives* 111 (2003): 1498-1504; James LeRoy et al., "Treatment Efficacy: A Survey of 305 MCS patients," *CFIDS Chronicle* (Winter 1996): 52-53; Alison Johnson, "Table of Survey Results from 351 Respondents." *MCS Information Exchange Newsletter*, September 19, 1997.

cannot go on living in a vehicle any longer & wonder if you know where I can turn to for help.

Some day I hope there will be an answer for desperate people like this woman. Now there is little, if anything, available to them. Mark, whose story appears in Part II, has lived in his car for over eleven years. And he is perfectly sane; I've met him on several occasions. You would not pick him out as a guy who has any problems, but his severe chemical sensitivity prevents him from working, and the disability check he receives is too small to enable him to pay for a housing situation that wouldn't involve sharing a house or apartment with roommates who would be using scented products or pesticides. Mark lives in a car because he's not ready to give up on life.

Chapter Three

The Consequences of Disbelief

One of the most difficult challenges faced by those with MCS is the widespread disbelief in the condition that they encounter from people who think it is simply a psychological disorder. Dr. Robert Haley of the University of Texas Southwestern Medical Center in Dallas, who is heading a $15 million-a-year research program on Gulf War syndrome, used to hold that opinion. When I was interviewing him for my book, *Gulf War Syndrome: Legacy of a Perfect War*, Dr. Haley told me: "Before I got involved in the Gulf War syndrome research, I assumed that MCS was a psychological problem. I've seen it now reported by so many veterans who clearly are not psychologically impaired that I now consider MCS and related problems a very serious medical issue in need of serious research" (p. 145).

The idea that chemical sensitivity is simply a psychological condition is illustrated by an article titled "Functional Somatic Syndromes" that appeared in *Annals of Internal Medicine* on June 1, 1999. In this article, Drs. Arthur J. Barsky and Jonathan F. Borus, psychiatrists at Brigham and Women's Hospital in Boston, stated: "The term functional somatic syndrome refers to several related syndromes that are characterized more by symptoms, suffering, and disability than by disease-specific, demonstrable abnormalities of structure or function." The authors note that physicians are "increasingly confronted by patients who have disabling, medically unexplained, somatic symptoms. . . . These patients often have a strong sense of assertiveness and embattled advocacy . . . And they may devalue and dismiss medical authority and epidemiologic evidence that conflicts with their beliefs."

Barsky and Borus's statement offers an excellent example of how people with chronic illnesses such as Gulf War syndrome, multiple chemical sensitivity, chronic fatigue syndrome, fibromyalgia, and sick building syndrome are viewed by physicians who do not like to have their authority questioned. These conditions, which many observers believe to be variants of the same underlying condition, are all listed in the Barsky and Borus article as examples of functional somatic syndromes. It is worth noting that Brigham and Women's Hospital, where Barsky and Borus work, was featured in a NOVA special on sick building syndrome that described how many nurses and other staff members of the hospital had developed chronic debilitating conditions like multiple chemical sensitivity. The hospital will have a substantial liability problem if multiple chemical sensitivity is recognized as a valid medical condition that can be precipitated by exposure to toxic chemicals.

Barsky and Borus's viewpoint is unfortunately held by many physicians and has contributed to an attitude of disbelief about chemical sensitivity among people such as landlords, employers, insurance companies, relatives, and friends, who affect in important ways the daily lives of those with MCS.

When I showed my *Toxic Clouds of 9/11* documentary in Ottawa in November 2006, a young woman in her twenties told me afterwards that she couldn't even spend Christmas with her family the next month. The reason? Her mother said they wouldn't be able to have a fire in the fireplace if she came. It seems likely that the mother thought her daughter's problems were imaginary and therefore did not deserve to be accommodated.

Disbelief was also a huge problem for Linda, who worked as a nurse in the VA state nursing home in Vermont. She developed MCS, as did four of her coworkers; they attributed their chemical sensitivity to the strong cleaning products used in the nursing home. When these women started asking their coworkers to refrain from wearing perfume, they were ostracized, as Linda describes in her story that appears in my book *Casualties of Progress*:

> Coworkers stopped speaking to us, and jokes were made at our expense. Then a new assistant administrator came on board who asked us if we were aware of internal e-mail messages that some of the women in the facility had been sending to one another about us on the company computers. . . .
>
> I find it hard to describe my emotions when I read the e-mail messages. I felt like I had been kicked in the stomach. . . .
> Reading how my coworkers conspired to wear heavy amounts of

perfume, all the same kind on the same day, was horrifying. They even named the day according to the perfume they chose to wear that day; for example, one day was named Peach Petals day.[1] They bragged about spraying the bathroom that we used with perfume and about spraying the top of the stairway that we used. They joked how all of us should dress up as "bubble people" for Halloween and they should dress up as cleaning products. One of the worst perfume offenders wrote on the e-mail, "like I said before, shoot the bitches. I know where we can get some bullets." And this woman is a registered nurse.

We did not obtain the e-mail messages until September 1996. It happened that my mother had died on July 15, 1996. I remember working on July 14, 1996, so ill I didn't think I could survive because the perfume was so heavy that day. The nursing home that my mother resided in called me on July 14 to tell me that she might not survive the night. My husband begged me to go to the emergency room for myself because I was having such a hard time breathing. My lungs were so congested that he could hear my respirations across the room. When I went home before going to be with my mom, my little girl said, "Mommy, you stink like perfume." My coworkers had worn so much perfume that day that I had absorbed it in my hair and clothing. But I couldn't take time to go to the emergency room because I wanted to be with my mother as she was dying. As it turned out, the nurses at her nursing home worried more about me that night than about their patients. I cannot forget how I suffered that night, both from losing my mom and from the physical suffering that I later learned was the result of a malicious prank by my coworkers. When I read the e-mail and recognized the date of Peach Petals day as being the day I was called to the nursing home to be with my dying mother, I felt violated. My grief felt fresh all over again.

Casualties of Progress, pp. 44-45

---

[1] Editor's note: To avoid possible liability, the real name of the perfume has not been used.

Because of the e-mail evidence, Linda was able to take her case to the Human Rights Commission of Vermont. In December 1996, its members voted in favor of her claim, stating that she had been discriminated against on the basis of a disability—MCS. I have heard of many similar cases, but I suspect that most people who hear about such abusive practices discount the reports, thinking that no one could be that mean. Sadly, the Vermont case indicates that even nurses can be cruel in some instances.

Unfortunately, the widespread disbelief about MCS in the medical community, which affects the attitudes of the general public, emboldens people like the nursing home employees who were in effect assaulting Linda and her sensitive coworkers with perfume. They may well have justified their bad behavior by a belief that Linda and the other women were just delusional people who were trying to control others in an unreasonable way.

Sp4c. Tara Batista, whose story appears in Part II, served as a medic and ambulance driver in the Gulf War and returned with a serious case of multiple chemical sensitivity. She encountered major problems with disbelief at the prison hospital in Massachusetts where she worked as a nurse.

A former marine who served in the Gulf War, S.Sgt. Terry Dillhyon, received a discharge summary from the VA hospital in Washington, D.C., that listed among his conditions "possible multiple chemical sensitivity." Terry reports in his story in Part II: "The doctor who told me I had multiple chemical sensitivity said he wasn't allowed to write that in the diagnosis—he could only say "possible multiple chemical sensitivity." The disbelief of a different physician had a huge financial impact on Terry, who is too sick to work and must use a wheelchair much of the time.

> When I went to a civilian doctor in connection with my application to obtain Medicare coverage from the Social Security Administration, I happened to mention that I had MCS. He went ballistic and said, "So you're one of those people. Let me tell you what, you just lost all your credibility with me." He turned in a negative report to the Social Security board, which then denied me Medicare coverage.

Not long after Terry was turned down for Medicare coverage, he ended up in the hospital because of an asthma attack precipitated by exposure to a perfume insert in a magazine he was reading. His ambulance, emergency room, and hospital bills totaled over $5,500, which Terry had to pay himself because he had been turned down for Medicare.

One of the sadder e-mails I recently received offers yet another example of the problems engendered by disbelief:

> I'm homeless in Washington DC. I reside in a homeless shelter that has no empathy for my chemical sensitivity. . . . The Staff at the shelter do not understand and do not take serious how ill I become when I have prolonged exposure to full strength bleach, pine sol, ammonia, aerosols.
>
> At times, the residents mix the chemicals together and also these chemicals are placed in pump-spray bottles and the residents spray these chemicals around the shelter just as you would air-freshener. Now that the residents know of this problem I have, just out of spite the residents just spray aerosols anytime most of the time when it is late at night and I can not leave the shelter for air. . . . I have spoken to staff about this and the issue, and of being assigned chores using these chemicals. The shelter director finds this issue a joke.

Joy, whose housing problem was described in Chapter 2, feels very isolated because of her children's attitudes toward multiple chemical sensitivity:

> After seven years of sharing information about my sickness with my children by sending videos, books, and articles, I found out they do not believe there is any such thing. My children and their spouses are in the medical profession. My son said that he is trying to understand, but everything I have sent is anecdotal with no medical proof. My daughter believes I am being "fed" symptoms, so that I believe I am ill. She is angry because I cannot travel 3,000 miles to visit. . . .
>
> Their disbelief has devastated me more than the disease itself. My children led me to believe they understood, but now I know they don't. I could take most of society believing it is "all in my head" but my own children!

> I thank the good Lord for a kind and understanding husband
> who respects me and knows how ill I get near chemicals and
> helps me so very much.
>
> *Casualties of Progress*, p. 209

One of Robert McCloskey's famous children's books, *One Morning in
Maine*, describes a morning spent taking his two little girls, Sal and
Jane, from the family island over to the mainland to buy supplies. The
setting seemed idyllic and pristine, but decades later, Jane, who was still
living in the same area of coastal Maine, developed multiple chemical
sensitivity. She too has had to struggle with disbelief:

> Over the years I have often experienced anger about how
> skeptics treated my MCS with contempt, skepticism, and a lack
> of compassion. Would the skepticism be overcome with time
> and truth, or would it remain forever? The answer, ten years
> later, is that many people are still skeptical and righteous in their
> disbelief. . . . Now I am resigned that without a research break-
> through, which doesn't seem likely, conventional doctors and
> those who trust them will continue to treat us with disbelief.
>
> *Casualties of Progress*, p. 198

Sue, who suffers from extreme chemical sensitivity, did give up on life
on two occasions, both directly related to the great difficulty she had
experienced trying to find a safe place to live and to work. In her story
in Part II, she describes in poignant terms the despair that drove her to
try to take her own life, even though she had a very supportive husband
who loved her very much. In her story, she relates the enormous sense
of frustration she felt when physicians, friends, and family viewed her
symptoms with skepticism.

One particularly tragic example of the fact that disbelief can indeed
sometimes kill appears in an e-mail that I recently received from Ann
McCampbell, M.D., a board member of the Chemical Sensitivity Foundation, who has written a very useful educational booklet on multiple
chemical sensitivity.[2] Dr. McCampbell wrote:

---

[2] See www.chemicalsensitivityfoundation.org, "Recommended Books and
Videos" section, for further information on Dr. McCampbell's booklet.

A woman, Rachel _____, had called me a couple weeks ago and wanted to order 50 of my booklets. When I called back to say they were ready to ship, a woman answered the phone and said that Rachel was "deceased," had hung herself about a week ago! How awful. She lived in Ohio.

I am wracking my brain to remember what she might have told me about her situation. I know she wanted booklets to try to increase awareness of and sympathy towards chemical sensitivities, but I don't remember the details.

It's clear that Rachel was so concerned about the disbelief she was encountering that she was willing to spend a considerable amount of money on booklets to try to counter this disbelief. Rachel's tragic death and Sue's two suicide attempts show that there are many ways to "assist" in suicide. Dr. Jack Kevorkian was strongly condemned for assisting in suicide. Unfortunately, many physicians, employers, family, and friends are in effect assisting in suicide through their disbelief.

In 1996, I happened to hear, somewhat by chance, that in the same three-week period that year two chemically sensitive people took their own lives and another woman with MCS ended up in the hospital with a failed suicide attempt. A number like this must unfortunately be only the tip of a dismaying iceberg. When I asked in my 1996 survey of 351 people with MCS if the respondents had heard of MCS suicides, I received reports of dozens of such suicides. One man replied:

Yes. It is fundamentally disturbing to me to relate that a very good friend of mine, a dear friend, committed suicide some few years ago. She was young, maybe 30. She was exquisitely sensitive and finding a reliably safe place for her to live was almost impossible. Her biggest problem though: No money except the minimum Social Security Income. Thoughts of her suicide still make my mind go numb. I myself will commit suicide sometime in the next few years. Why? Too maladaptive with no money as offset.

Casualties of Progress, pp. 145-46

About five years after this man wrote this passage, I met him when I was traveling on the West Coast. He is a very intelligent, reasonable, and likable person who is doing his best to stay alive, and I hope he does.

One sometimes hears reporters or people in the medical profession say somewhat glibly that no one ever dies of multiple chemical sensitivity. Would these same people say that no one ever dies from bipolar disease, which has a significant mortality rate from suicide?

Twelve years as an advocate for the chemically sensitive has led me to the sad realization that a large number of chemically sensitive people have taken their own lives and many others are inching ever closer to that decision because they find it such a daunting task to locate a safe place to live or work and are rapidly running out of money. And at the same time that they are engaged in this herculean struggle, far too many of them are facing a discouraging skepticism from those about them.

What can people who are lucky enough not to have developed MCS do to ameliorate this tragic situation? Keeping an open mind and a compassionate attitude would be a good first step. An overview of the subject of MCS is available on the website of the Chemical Sensitivity Foundation, www.chemicalsensitivityfoundation.org. That website also contains a long bibliography of research studies on chemical sensitivity that have been published in peer-reviewed journals. Even just skimming that bibliography should dispel the notion that there is no scientific evidence that MCS is a physiologically based medical condition. (This twelve-page research bibliography, which includes studies from not only the United States, but also Japan, Denmark, Germany, Greece, Spain, Italy, and Sweden, also appears on pp. 289-300 of this book.)

Physicians and nurses need to educate themselves more about the condition of chemical sensitivity, so that MCS patients can get more help from the mainstream medical community. At present, disbelief among many physicians has the outcome that many chemically sensitive people seek out alternative medicine practitioners. The latter are helpful in many cases, but there are also many people in this group who are taking advantage of the desperate plight of people with multiple chemical sensitivity.

It is particularly important that psychiatrists, psychologists, and social workers begin to understand that MCS is indeed a medically valid diagnosis and not just a quaint and annoying delusion of patients who are paranoid about chemicals in the modern world. When professionals in these fields view MCS patients as being delusional and paranoid because they report that chemical exposures are causing them to develop various symptoms, the consequences can be extreme. There have been many cases in which family members or neighbors of MCS patients have attempted, sometimes successfully, to have them admitted to mental hospitals for no reason but their belief that they are suffering from multiple chemical sensitivity.

Some professionals in this field as well as members of the general public have gone so far as to suggest that parents who have children with MCS are "creating" this illness in their children in order to obtain attention from the medical community. These skeptics are suggesting that what is involved in these chemical sensitivity cases is a rare syndrome that has been termed "Munchausen by Proxy" in which a parent actually inflicts minor injuries on a child because they enjoy the resultant medical attention. The mother of an eight-year-old boy named Zack, who developed severe chemical sensitivity following a furnace explosion when he was a baby, faced this kind of accusation:

> People tend to be skeptical about Zack's illness and look for other explanations for whatever is wrong with him. After an article about Zack appeared in the local newspaper, some woman went to the school and handed one of the administrators an article on Munchausen by Proxy.
>
> *Casualties of Progress*, p. 77

Christi Howarth is a single mother with a twelve-year-old son who almost lost her son in a court battle with California's Child Protective Services. She had been a teacher in the California system for over twenty-five years, with a specialty in teaching gifted children. Unfortunately, Christi and her son both developed MCS in their adjacent school buildings located a block from the ocean. She reports that there were mold problems in both schools, her building had ongoing gas leaks, and contaminated soil was removed from the site of the schools. Blood tests showed benzene in her blood and xylene in her son's blood. Christi went to some highly respected physicians in the field of chemical injury and mold exposures and has extensive documentation for her and her son's health conditions. Their chemical sensitivity is severe enough that she can no longer teach and he cannot attend school. He would develop migraine headaches, breathing difficulty, extreme fatigue, and nose bleeds in his school building. He has been diagnosed with asthma, and his symptoms now include facial tics and rashes upon exposure to various chemicals. Christi finally decided to home school him, and his symptoms have diminished with the reduced exposures.

An ophthalmologist who saw Christi was concerned because she had inflamed eyelids and recommended that she consult an infectious disease specialist. Christi decided to include her son in the appointment because his eyelids were similarly inflamed. To her dismay, the specialist whom she consulted was totally dismissive of the records Christi brought along that documented chemical sensitivity and mold reactions in her and her son. In fact, she immediately reported Christi to the Child Protective Services, saying that she was delusional about her son's health problems. That started a nightmare for Christi, who was forced to spend almost all her savings to fight a difficult legal battle. And Christi was alone in this fight; she was raised by her grandparents, now deceased, and her son's father is not in the picture. Christi not only had no one to help her financially, she also was devastated to think that her son, who is the only family she has, could be taken away from her and put into foster care.

Her son was also traumatized by the whole affair. What could be more terrifying to a twelve-year-old boy than to think that he is about to be taken away from his mother, who is the only family he has? Life with a foster family, who would have almost certainly been instructed by Child Protective Services to ignore his delusion about chemical sensitivity, would have been an impossible nightmare for this child.

Fortunately, Christi finally prevailed in the court system, and the court procedures to allow Child Protective Services to assume custody of her son were terminated, but not without a crushing financial cost to Christi. In an appalling aftermath of the whole nightmare, Christi's name was listed on an index of child abusers after the initial visit she received from a social worker from Child Protective Services, who thought Christi's medical beliefs were delusional. This means that if she recovers her health sufficiently to be able to teach school again, no school system will hire her. Her legal counsel has advised her that it is a very difficult and costly procedure to have one's name removed from the index of child abusers once it has been placed there.

A little time spent by individuals who are not chemically sensitive to educate themselves about the field will have an important effect on the lives of many desperate people like Christi. And such increased awareness of chemical sensitivity may even produce unexpected health benefits for those who have never pondered the issue.

Chapter 4

The EPA Headquarters
Becomes a Sick Building

It seemed a minor event when the EPA began to install about 27,000 square yards of carpet in hundreds of offices in its new headquarters building in the Waterside Mall in Washington, D.C., in 1987. But the federal agency charged with protecting our environment was about to impact its own indoor air quality in a major way and make hundreds of its employees sick. Many would never recover their health.

At that time, the EPA was a relatively new federal agency, having been created by Congress in 1977. After limping along for ten years in temporary quarters, the agency needed a permanent home and was persuaded to sign a twenty-year lease on the Waterside Mall, even though it had been designed as a shopping mall, not for office space.

It's hardly surprising that the conversion of a shopping mall into an office building did not yield optimal results. There were, of course, virtually no windows in the building. The larger spaces of retail stores were chopped up into a virtual rabbit warren of small offices with no windows. James Handley, an attorney with a chemistry background who started working at the EPA in 1987, never forgot his first day in the building, when his new boss, John Wheeler, showed him around:

> My first visit to the EPA headquarters in the Waterside Mall in southwest Washington left an indelible impression: the building is one of the most dreary, depressing, and ugly places I've ever set foot in. Wheeler escorted me down winding corridors that were so narrow that two people could barely pass. These hallways were dimly lit by flickering blue flourescent lights and were punctuated by missing ceiling tiles and stacks of worn-out office equipment, boxes, and other junk. A stale, vaguely chemical odor hung in the air.
>
> Part II, p. 116

Bobbie Lively-Diebold, a senior scientist at the EPA, recounts what happened to her in the Waterside Mall on a day that would change her life forever:

> Early in the morning on January 22, 1988, soon after the renovation had begun and the new carpet had been installed, I entered my office and smelled a strong, acrid chemical smell. Almost immediately, I began coughing and felt dizzy and nauseated. My breathing became labored, and I experienced pain in my lungs. In addition, I became disoriented and lost my voice. I left the office and remained outside until my head was clear enough that I could drive home.
>
> Part II, p. 173

After Bobbie had spent a few days at home, her supervisor allowed her to try working in various other sections of the Waterside Mall where carpet had not yet been installed. Unfortunately, Bobbie also became sick in the other areas of the building, probably because the HVAC (heating/ventilation/air conditioning system) was circulating the fumes from the remodeling throughout the building. Because of these troubling symptoms, Bobbie's doctor helped her obtain workers' compensation so she could stay out of the Waterside Mall for six weeks. Although her symptoms diminished during this period, they returned in full force when she went back to work, as she describes:

> I returned from lunch one day to find that carpet was being installed in an area several hundred feet away from our section. Shortly after I entered the building, I had an even stronger attack than the initial one I had experienced in January. I gasped for breath, my lungs burned, my face turned bright red, and my heartbeat became irregular. I was confused and disoriented, and I couldn't talk. Someone helped me to an elevator, and I stumbled outside the building. Unable to walk, I sat down on the ground next to a pillar in the rain. Some of the people who walked by asked me if something was wrong and if they could help me. I stayed in the rain for a long time too dazed to do or say anything. Somehow I managed to get home, and that was the last time I entered the Waterside Mall.
>
> Part II, p. 175

Over a decade later I met Bobbie Lively-Diebold when I showed my MCS video to a group of chemically sensitive people who had gathered in the home of another EPA scientist who had become sick and had developed multiple chemical sensitivity during the renovation. Partway through the showing, Bobbie started reacting to something in her friend's living room and had to excuse herself. I slipped out into the hall to say good-bye to her and her husband, but just as I was shaking her hand, Bobbie began having muscle spasms. She started lurching all around the hall with my hand tightly held in hers. Finally, her husband was able to pry her fingers loose from my hand. That was an unforgettable example of the neurological damage that has occurred in some chemically sensitive people.

In her story in Part II, Bobbie describes the chemical sensitivity she developed after exposure to the toxic EPA carpet:

> Perfume and scented products made me violently ill. I could not pump gas for my car or do many of the tasks of everyday life that most people take for granted. Walking down the grocery aisle where soaps and cleaning products were displayed made me quite ill. . . . When I was in a car, I had to wear a respirator containing charcoal cartridges to protect myself from the traffic exhaust. I sometimes had episodes at a doctor's office where exposures in that atmosphere would cause one of my arms to start shaking violently or I would become nauseated or feel very ill. Somewhere along the line, the folks in our COPE [Committee of Poisoned Employees] group did research and found that there was a name for our condition–multiple chemical sensitivity (MCS).

Bobbie was not the only EPA employee who was reacting to the fumes from the new carpet. More and more people were heading to the EPA Health Unit to complain that they were being sickened by the new carpet and paint fumes associated with the remodeling. Mark Bradley, M.D., an occupational medicine physician working in the health unit, reported the following results to EPA Administrator William Reilly:

> At least 80% of the [approximately 60] individuals who I examined, have bone fide medical problems which I believe are caused by working at the Waterside Mall complex. Fifty to sixty percent

had symptoms and physical findings . . . typical of "Tight Building Syndrome" . . . eye and throat irritation, headaches . . . some people were severely affected. Thirty to forty percent . . . had symptoms of airway hyperreactivity . . . a form of occupational asthma. Ten percent of patients had evidence of allergic alveolitis, an inflammatory reaction in the alveoli and bronchioles of the lung resulting from an immune interaction between inhaled organic particles, circulating antibodies and sensitized lymphocites [*sic*]. This condition can be progressive, leading to progressive pulmonary impairment and death. . . . I am certain that . . . I saw only a small fraction of the people . . . potentially adversely affected. . . . There is a major public health situation at this location, and . . .[it] is not being dealt with in a timely, positive and responsible fashion.

Part II, p. 121

As James Handley notes in his story in Part II, "The EPA's response to Dr. Bradley (a contract employee) was to immediately terminate his employment."

One of the employees whose health was severely impacted by the toxic air that was circulating through the building was an attorney who had worked at the EPA headquarters since 1984 in the Office of Enforcement. She wrote the following account of her experience:

The first life-threatening crisis I faced was in mid-August of 1988. That morning I left my air-conditioned home and car pooled in an air-conditioned car to the underground garage at the Waterside Mall. After spending about thirty minutes in my air-conditioned office, I began to feel weak and light-headed. I walked over to the EPA Health Unit and almost passed out when I got to the door. I remember the nurse talking to me, shaking me gently, and telling me not to go to sleep. She asked me if I had any chest pains, but I didn't. All I had was a sense of darkness closing in around me and deep fatigue. I remember hearing the nurse tell a doctor that my pulse was 42 and my blood pressure was something just over 50. The next thing I remember is being in an ambulance on the way to the emergency room at George Washington Hospital. Curiously, when I later asked for all the records of my visits to the EPA Health Unit for my lawsuit, there was a conspicuous gap. My August collapse in the building was missing.

The George Washington ER doctor put me on oxygen and released me when my heart rate got up to 50 or so. Strangely enough, the diagnosis on the ER report was "heat exhaustion," despite the fact that I had spent the whole day in air-conditioned places.

When I described what had happened that day during a follow-up visit with a doctor at George Washington Hospital, she assured me that there was nothing wrong with the Waterside Mall. She even suggested that I was unhappy with my job. Even so, she gave me a prescription for oxygen on demand to use at the EPA Health Unit. I became a regular visitor there in the weeks to come. One time when I went in for oxygen, the nurse said they were out. When I asked her how many other EPA employees were coming in for oxygen, she said she was not allowed to give out that information.

Part II, p. 261

The EPA employees who were developing serious health problems turned for help to the union that represented the EPA's professional employees, the National Federation of Federal Employees, Local 2050. One of its officers, Bill Hirzy, a Ph.D. chemist who later became president of the union, became very actively involved in attempting to protect the rights of the sick workers and worked closely with James Handley, who served as the union's secretary.

The union published articles about the carpet problem in its newsletter and urged employees who were having health problems to report to the EPA Health Unit. The union's health and safety representatives soon learned that the ventilation system in the Waterside Mall was not bringing in enough fresh air. Most of the air coming out of the vents in each office was recycled air, some of it from rooms full of xerox machines that were in almost constant use. James Handley noticed that he could hear the ventilation blowers shut down late in the afternoon. When he investigated, he found that the maintenance man in charge was turning off the blowers when he left for the day, sometimes as early as 3:30 P.M., despite the fact that the EPA flex-time workday didn't end until 7 P.M.

By this point, the EPA was feeling pressure not only from the union but also from the media. Ed Bradley interviewed Bill Hirzy and James Handley on CBS's "Street Stories," and Bobbie Lively-Diebold spoke out on "Good Morning America," "Larry King Live," the "Today Show," and "60 Minutes." The media jumped on the irony that the EPA, which was supposed to be protecting all Americans from toxic exposures, couldn't even get it right in its own national headquarters building. Under constant pressure from the union, the EPA finally agreed to remove all the carpet from its headquarters building. Unfortunately, its employees had been breathing the fumes from this carpet for almost two years.

To compound the air quality problems in the Waterside Mall, the lack of proper ventilation with an adequate fresh air intake exacerbated not only the problem of the carpet fumes but also the problem of the noxious fumes from a roofing operation begun in September 1990 to replace the flat asphalt roof of the three-story mall building, as James Handley notes:

> One day another attorney and I were at a meeting on the fifth floor of the West Tower. From that vantage point, we could see below us the roof of the mall, where the roofing work was being done over our offices. We could see the caldrons of tar with the gray vapor rising a few feet and then curling back down as it was sucked into the building through a nearby air intake. The pungent, sulfurous smell of tar permeated our offices for months. Thick, gray smoke frequently impaired the visibility in the corridors and offices. Inhaling the smoke made my head ache and my chest tighten, as if someone were sitting on me, so it was a struggle to breathe.
>
> Part II, pp. 122-23

The strong fumes from the tar caught up with James Handley on February 25, 1991, a day when they were especially thick. While he was participating in a conference call in his supervisor's office, James passed out. His shocked supervisor at that point urged him to pursue the option of working from home, which he decided to do.

James Handley continued to work with union president Bill Hirzy to call the attention of Congress to toxicity issues with new carpet. Their efforts culminated in several hearings, including one held by the Senate Oversight Committee on Governmental Affairs on October 1, 1992. At this hearing, Bill Hirzy testified about his attempts to draft a plan with the EPA leaders to investigate possible toxicity issues with new carpet in general:

> At this point the light came on for me–it appeared that EPA would not participate in activities that would place the carpet industry at risk from tort actions . . .
>
> . . . . .
>
> In January 1990, despairing of effective initiatives by EPA management, the union filed a petition under section 21 of TSCA [Toxic Substance Control Act] asking EPA to take regulatory action. EPA denied the petition, telling the union "off the record" that it would not grant the petition because it would cost the carpet industry "billions of dollars."

Bill Hirzy also submitted to the Senate committee a summary of the efforts by the attorneys general of twenty-six states to investigate the issue of new carpet toxicity, efforts that were necessitated by the lack of attention that the EPA was giving this important issue.

At a hearing of the House Oversight Committee for Governmental Affairs held on June 11, 1993, toxicologist Rosalind Anderson, who holds a Ph.D. degree from Yale, testified about a neurotoxic chemical called 4-phenylcyclohexane that she had found in the EPA carpet samples. Dr. Anderson then showed a video of an experiment she had performed that illustrated the devastating effects that exposure to the EPA carpet samples had upon mice.

Despite the various congressional hearings held on the carpet issue, the EPA refused to take any action to protect the general public from toxic carpets and also refused to compensate its sick employees. Five EPA employees who became chronically ill after exposure to the toxic carpet at the EPA headquarters finally started a lawsuit against the owners of the Waterside Mall building in 1992. When the case went to trial years later, the jury gave the employees low monetary awards, but the judge tried to deny those awards. His decision was eventually overturned, and the case was settled out of court in 2001.

In the meantime, the EPA continued through the 1990s to deny any responsibility for the sharp decline in the health of a large number of its employees who were exposed to the carpet installed in 1987, and the agency resolutely refused to concede that these employees had developed chemical sensitivity as a result of this exposure. Thus the EPA let slip a historic opportunity to understand the issue of chemical sensitivity, and many people across the country–their ranks include *Exxon Valdez* cleanup workers, Gulf War veterans, 9/11 First Responders, and Katrina victims–would ultimately see their health and lives wrecked as a result of the EPA's political decision to protect the carpet industry and to deny the reality of multiple chemical sensitivity.

Chapter 5

The *Exxon Valdez* Cleanup

When the *Exxon Valdez* tanker ran aground in late March 1989 on a reef in the Alaskan paradise of Prince William Sound, it spread an ominous stain of more than 10 million gallons of crude oil over the pristine waters and the beaches surrounding the huge bay. The oil spill was immediately recognized as a cataclysmic event of vast implications for the ecology of one of the most remote and beautiful spots in the world. In 1989 attention was focused on the health of the sea vegetation and aquatic birds and mammals, but the way the cleanup was handled would have devastating consequences for the health of the people who were hired to help in the attempt to remove the oil from the beaches.

As the news of the largest oil spill in U.S. history quickly spread to every corner of the globe, Exxon knew at once that it was facing a public relations disaster of epic proportions. Exxon officials rushed to Alaska to put in place a massive containment and cleanup operation. And just as quickly as the Exxon officials started pouring into the port of Valdez, an army of reporters and photographers began arriving to document this ecological disaster that was instantly recognized to be one of the environmental stories of the century.

Exxon was not in an enviable position because it quickly became known that the *Valdez* captain was intoxicated when he ran his huge tanker aground on Bligh Reef. Worse yet for the beleaguered oil giant, it turned out that company officials were well aware of Captain Joe Hazelwood's drinking problem.

Under the spotlight of media attention, Exxon knew that it must act as fast as possible to remove the remaining oil from the grounded ship and to clean the beaches that had already been covered with the sticky black mass.

Seeing not only their beloved waterways but also their future liveli-hood at risk, the men and women who captained fishing boats rushed to the scene within hours of the disaster to do what they could to help contain the oil spill until enough larger vessels could arrive to off-load the *Exxon Valdez*'s huge cargo of oil. Unfortunately, before the larger vessels brought in by Exxon could pump the remaining oil out of the leaking hold onto other vessels, nature dealt a huge blow to these efforts. Three days after the intoxicated captain of the *Exxon Valdez* let it run aground, there was a massive storm whose high winds and powerful waves quickly pushed the oil slick onto the far-flung beaches that dotted the islands and the perimeter of Prince William Sound.

The media feeding frenzy was a major factor driving Exxon to move as quickly as possible to mitigate a public relations nightmare. One of Exxon's first moves was to subcontract the job of cleaning up the oil-covered beaches to a company called VECO. By April, VECO had hired thousands of workers. Ultimately about eleven thousand people worked in the cleanup operation in various ways, most of them on the beaches, with others manning boats that placed booms and skimmed up oil washed off the beaches. The people who worked on the beaches were housed in berthing barges from which they would travel by smaller boats each day to the beach where they were assigned. The hours were grueling; most workers report having worked twelve-hour shifts (not including travel time), seven days a week. Thus their bodies had little chance to recuperate from the various toxins to which they were being exposed. They were allowed to take time off every so often, but many found that a two- or three-day leave was hardly practical since they would use up much of it traveling back and forth to their homes.

One man hired to help in the cleanup was a construction worker named Robert Bunker, who describes in his story in Part II the difficult working conditions on the beaches:

All day long we were wallowing in oil. We were falling down all the time. I screwed up my knees real bad slipping on all those oily rocks, and I still have lots of pain in my knees. It was very bad; the rocks were kind of like bowling balls covered with oil. It was a big slippery mess. After the first few days, I was having nightmares that I was drowning in oil.

Part II, p. 190

Phyllis "Dolly" LaJoie, who worked first on a decontamination area of a berthing barge and later on the beaches, remembers the overpowering odor on the beaches:

> The smell on the beaches was awful, like something dead. Crude oil has a sickening odor all its own. It's horrible. Of course, there were dead things, too . . . We would put the dead seals or birds in plastic bags. It was pretty sickening to have to pick up these animals and birds that had been decomposing for several months.
>
> Part II, pp. 245-46

VECO's plan for cleaning the beaches evolved during the first few days. Initially, workers were given "pom-poms," so named because the bunches of strands of absorbent material resemble a cheerleader's pom-pom. During these early days, the plan was to have the workers wipe the oil off the rocks with these absorbent pom-poms, which would then be put into plastic bags for transport elsewhere. Of course, it didn't take too many days for the futility of such an effort to become apparent, although this method continued to be used in a limited way. Greta, a beach worker who developed chemical sensitivity after working on the oil spill, describes what it was like to try to clean the oil off the rocks with pom-poms:

> We would sit down on the rocks while we were working because it was hard to bend down for hour after hour. There were fumes coming off the oily rocks, and between the rocks there were puddles of oil containing decaying seaweed that smelled really bad. I remember a couple of spots that smelled so terrible that we could only work there for a few minutes at a time. People were getting light-headed and dizzy and nauseous from the oil fumes; we sometimes felt like we might pass out. They had to take one person off the beach because she was starting to hallucinate.
>
> . . . . . .
>
> We were always sitting in oil, and the odor would give us headaches. When we leaned down to work, oil would often splatter on our faces and sometimes our wrists would get exposed. We couldn't pull off our gloves to eat without ending up with oil on our hands and on our food. After you pulled off

one glove, you had to pull the other glove off with your bare hand, so of course you ended up with oil all over that hand.

Part II, pp. 115-16

VECO's next plan was to wash the oil off the rocks and beaches onto the edge of the bay, catch it with booms, and then skim it up into boats to be shipped elsewhere. Streams of water from large high-pressure hoses were used to dislodge the oil from the rocky beaches. Crews soon discovered that hot water would pull more of the oil off the rocks, so hot water was used whenever possible. Steam guns were also used to steam the oil off the rocks.

In her book *Sound Truth and Corporate Myth$: The Legacy of the Exxon Valdez Oil Spill,* Dr. Riki Ott, a marine biologist from Cordova, Alaska, notes that many observers questioned the advisability of the steam and hot water operation:

> NOAA [National Oceanographic and Atmospheric Association] scientists also warned that the pressurized hot water wash was cooking beach life and killing the few hardy plants and animals that had survived the initial oiling. . . . With no survivors to recolonize and restore life, NOAA scientists warned that the "treated" beaches might actually take longer to recover than beaches that were left alone.
>
> . . . .
>
> Coast Guard Vice Admiral Clyde Robbins, the person ultimately responsible for approving the steam cleaning and overseeing the cleanup, asked, "How much damage do you want to do to a beach to save it? I don't want people to say about me that I killed Alaska trying to save it."

(Ott, p. 31)

The steam and hot water were a problem not only for the plants and marine animals on the beaches but also for the cleanup workers. Unfortunately, both the steam from the steam guns and the hot water from the high-pressure hoses created an oily mist that the workers were inhaling and getting on their faces and in their eyes. Regrettably, government agencies that should have protected the workers from this exposure did not do their job. In a statement that is eerily reminiscent of Christine Todd Whitman's declaration to New Yorkers a few days after 9/11 that their air was "safe to breathe," the Alaska Department of Health and Social Services issued an advisory stating:

> There is no risk of adverse health effects from breathing the air. Risks are greatest to workers heavily exposed to oil during some cleanup activities, but the risks to these workers is considered to be low and with appropriate training and personal protective equipment as required by the hazardous waste regulations, clean-up activities can continue and workers can be confident that their health will not be compromised.
>
> (Ott, p. 27)

On the beaches in Alaska as in the rubble and smoke near Ground Zero, personal protective equipment was in short supply and even though the Occupational Safety and Health Act (OSHA) should have protected the workers in Prince William Sound and Lower Manhattan, that was not the case.

Some workers survived their exposures in Prince William Sound with no apparent health effects; others were not so lucky, as is indicated by the stories of three brothers who cleaned the Alaska beaches and three scientists who traveled from California to study the cleanup process so that their state could be better prepared for its next oil spill.

The Potter brothers–Roger, Mike, and Paul–were construction workers who had been having trouble finding enough work after the Alaskan pipeline was finished, so they quickly signed on to help in the cleanup operation. A picture of Roger clad in an oily rain outfit and wearing no respirator as he steams oil off rocks appears on the cover of Riki Ott's book. He was the lucky one of the three brothers. During the first couple of months he was working on the oil spill, he did develop some brown blisters on his lower legs that would pop and ooze a brown liquid, but they were gone by November. At this point, he doesn't think that his work on the spill affected his health in any lasting way.

His brother Mike was not so lucky, as he recounts in the story of the Potter brothers that appears in Part II:

> We felt nauseated all the time we were working out there on the beaches, and headaches were rampant. . . . Then in addition to all the oil we were exposed to, there were a bunch of chemicals that we used. We would request and request that we be

given the hazardous chemical plat that was supposed to be on top of the containers of chemicals, but we never could find out what ingredients were in the containers. We didn't have more than a name on the container. . . . We nicknamed one chemical Agent Orange. One of the things it was used for was to wash the oil off the boats and skiffs. It was eating the membranes in people's noses. On our second or third R&R, word was getting out that if you are asked to work around this chemical, you should refuse to do it.

. . . . . .

I started having some fairly serious memory loss problems a few years after the spill, even though I was only in my thirties. People would say, "Mike, how are you doing?" and I wouldn't recognize them. I used to know the phone numbers of people I call a lot. Now I have to look them up.

   I developed some growths that looked like a huge wart. They were 3/4" thick and about the size of a silver dollar. Those big wart-like growths appeared about three years after I had worked on the oil-spill cleanup. A lot of my ailments started around 1993. That was when I started having some black-out spells and getting serious fatigue.

                                        Part II, pp. 150-51

Eventually Mike's health problems made it necessary for him to give up construction work and become a mechanic. Even in that job he found that his arthritis was made worse by some of the cleaning solvents that he had to use.

   Chemical sensitivity was an even greater problem for the youngest brother, Paul, as Mike recounts:

We were picking up debris like dead oil-soaked wildlife that gave off a terrible rotten stench. We put this stuff in plastic bags to be picked up by a little barge, and these bags were sitting on the beaches in the hot sun. Usually the tops were twisted, but when Paul picked up this one bag, the top swirled open and gases poured out onto his face. He staggered around and said he couldn't see, so some guys had to grab him. They sent him to Anchorage on a helicopter, and he spent several days in a hospital there. The exposure kind of paralyzed his breathing. He got some of the stuff in one of his eyes and almost lost it; he was actually blind for a while. . . . After that incident, almost any chemical would cause Paul to feel nauseated.

Part II, p. 151

According to Paul's widow, after he stopped working on the oil-spill cleanup, products that he had regularly used in his carpentry work started bothering him:

There were at least four times that he had to get medical attention because of exposure to something toxic. One time when he was putting a sealant on a deck, he got really sick and dizzy, so they had to take him to a clinic. They called a poison hot line and hooked him up to IVs to get him stabilized. Sometimes he would have a milder reaction, but he would still end up stuck in bed for a couple of days with a violent headache, feeling yucky and kind of weak. He would react to almost anything that was petroleum based. Once when we were painting an apartment and using an oil-based primer on the walls, he almost passed out into the tray of paint. He had never reacted to things like that before *Exxon Valdez*. . . .

At the time Paul died, the two of us were working as caretakers for an apartment complex. The week before he died he told me that the gas fumes from the snow blower were starting to make him sick. After he told me that the gas fumes from the snow blower were beginning to bother him, I tried to get him to let me do all the snow blowing around the apartments. It was the man-thing though–he wouldn't let me do it. It was only a half hour after he came in from snow blowing one day that he had a massive heart attack. He died in the ambulance on the way to the hospital. His doctor said that the snow blower gas fumes were most likely what had killed him. Paul was only forty-four when he died.

Part II, pp. 151-52

Among the results of the intense public focus on how quickly the oil was being dispersed was Exxon's dubious decision to use chemical dispersants on the oil-covered beaches, a decision that led to some serious toxic exposures for the three scientists from California.

Bob Curry was part of this scientific team that traveled to Prince William Sound from the Monterey, California, area, where he taught geology at the University of California at Santa Cruz. One member of the team was a former physician, one was a marine biologist, and Bob was a geologist in the field of water quality. Bob had at one point in his life taught at the University of Alaska and was particularly interested in the marine food chain, including whales. The three scientists were especially interested in learning how California might minimize the damage to marine life if there were another oil spill like the one that had occurred near Santa Barbara. They traveled around Prince William Sound in their own small boat, filming the cleanup crews on beaches and trying to evaluate the effectiveness of the various cleanup methods.

They went ashore on a number of islands and peninsulas and usually camped on the beaches. One of Bob's projects was to dig pits on the beaches to analyze how much oil lay below the surface of the beach, ready to be released in a storm. In some places they learned that the beach crews were using Corexit, a chemical about which Bob and his teammates knew nothing at first. Then they met with Alaska state officials who said it was important to be very careful around this chemical. The officials showed them labels saying that one should have no skin contact and should not breathe the fumes, but the latter injunction seemed hard to carry out because the chemical was being sprayed on the beaches. The workers who were applying the Corexit were wearing chemical suits, but the cleanup workers who followed them in a day or two, like Bob and his colleagues, had no protective gear.

In all, the three scientists spent seven days working on the beaches. At the time, they experienced no effects, but ten days after they had returned to California, Bob developed a severe respiratory problem that resembled pneumonia. When it persisted, he began to wonder if his fairly extensive handling of Corexit-contaminated sand could have caused his illness. He found out that the marine biologist who had gone to Prince William Sound with him had also become sick shortly after returning but had recovered in a week, whereas Bob Curry had been sick at that point for over a month with a pneumonia-like illness.

Finally, after six months, Bob Curry was able to shake off the problem in his lungs, which physicians had never been able to diagnose. Although Bob Curry was able to get rid of his pneumonia-like lung problem, he developed acute asthma not long after he returned from Alaska and now gets an asthma attack from exposure to all sorts of chemicals.

Unfortunately, Bob has in the last several years developed a very serious health problem, as he noted in an e-mail he recently sent me:

> I have now been diagnosed with rather pronounced brain atrophy that the neurologists suggest must be chemically caused. I am now being probed, spinal-tapped and chemically assessed to try to find out what could have caused it. Because I am now seventy-one and the Prince William Sound Corexit exposure was long ago, I have little confidence that anything will be found. But the neurologists say that the changes are dramatic and progressive and must be chemically induced. Symptoms at first were a staggering gait and movement disorders indicating cerebellar ataxia resulting from the MRI-verified cerebellar atrophy. Now the primary concern is loss of more of the primary brain.
>
> Based on movement disorders that became serious in about 2002 and lack of ability to maintain balance, I first had a series of CAT scans and then recently have had a series of MRIs. These various scans show progressive atrophy of the whole brain that is not caused by local strokes or accidents or any direct causes except possible past chemical exposure. Present symptoms are like some aspects of Parkinson's Disease, but these symptoms are not the result of losses of only that part of the basal brain stem and/or cerebellum involved in Parkinson's Disease.

Betty Blankenship also had a heavy exposure to various chemicals used during the two summers she worked on the cleanup operation. One of her jobs was to wash boats that were coated with oil, a process that entailed the use of strong solvents. Much of her work was done inside the boats, where the solvent fumes had less chance to dissipate. Her husband Robert reports another exposure that was particularly trouble-some. During most of one summer, Betty spent seven to twelve hours a day working in a containment pit where they mixed up chemicals. She told her husband that she saw chemical barrels that had a skull and crossbones on them. She wore a protective full-body suit but said that many people were not wearing these protective suits. According to Robert, Betty reported that people were getting holes in their rubber boots and heavy-duty rain gear within a few days of working around these chemicals.

One day Betty had to go to the emergency room for a respiratory problem, where her blood was tested for six gases. Robert reports that she was asked to sign some paper at the ER and was never given the results of the tests for various gases. After the cleanup, she suffered from respiratory problems, an irregular heartbeat, and thyroid problems.

Betty died in May 2001 at the age of forty-one, leaving children aged ten, fourteen, seventeen, and twenty. Robert initially thought she had died of cardiac arrest, but a doctor he talked to shortly after she died said that she had probably died of arrhythmia.

The chemicals that were used in connection with the spill cleanup were also a big factor in the problems that Dolly LaJoie developed after working on the spill. Her health deteriorated sharply after she finished working on the oil spill cleanup, but years later she not only had to put up with failing health that made it impossible for her to keep working but was also told by one physician that she was a hypochondriac with no real health problems. It was clear to me in the phone interviews I did with Dolly that she was a very sick woman. She was coughing so badly from her asthma during our first conversation that I had to suggest that I call her back in a few days.

Dolly's story in Part II details her widespread exposures to toxins during her work on the beaches and in the decontamination unit where she worked for twelve hours every night for several weeks to remove the oil from the beach workers' clothing, boots, and gloves.

> We washed the oily coveralls and underwear in the washing machine. We used Tide at first, but then they started sending us some strong solvents to add because it was really hard to get the oil out of everything. . . . It was industrial strength stuff. I don't remember all the names, but one product we used was Simple Green. The laundry room, which held just one washer and dryer, was small, and the vapor made me sick a lot of the time. When you washed the oily clothes and dried them in the

dryer, you had oil vapor everywhere, and it was a strong smell. Sometimes I felt like I was drunk and felt like I was going to pass out. I would have to go outside to get away from the fumes and get some fresh air. Whenever it was really cold, as it often was at night, we would have to keep the laundry room door shut to keep from freezing, and then the fumes were really thick.

Part II, pp. 244

Simple Green, the product to which Dolly was exposed in the laundry room, along with crude oil, was one of many industrial-strength solvents that cleanup workers used. According to the Material Safety Data Sheet for this product, it contains 2-butoxyethanol. The EPA website that offers guidance on janitorial products lists the following chronic effects from 2-butoxyethanol: "Reproductive & Fetal Effects; Liver & Kidney Damage; Blood Damage" and includes this warning:

> If at all possible, avoid janitorial products with the following ingredients [the table includes 2-butoxyethanol]. They pose very high risks to the janitor using the product, to building occupants, or to the environment.

Dolly, like the other *Exxon Valdez* cleanup workers whose stories are included in Part II, has been left with a troubling legacy of chemical sensitivity, as she notes: "Traffic exhaust gives me a headache and makes me nauseated. Cigarette smoke and certain cleaning products and perfumes make me choke and cough, give me a headache, and make me sick to my stomach." Greta too is now chemically sensitive: "I always end up with a headache if I use hair spray, and I can't use perfume now because it gives me a headache and often makes me feel angry. I have to avoid gasoline and diesel. My parents and my sister who worked the spill with me can't use perfume now either, and we all have to be very careful what cleaning products we use." Chemical exposures are also now a serious problem for Robert Bunker: "I get bad headaches and real shaky when I'm around gasoline or paint fumes or smoke."

What is particularly striking about the *Exxon Valdez* situation is the immense disparity between the plight of the people who ruined their health working on the cleanup and the tremendous wealth of Exxon (now ExxonMobil). Given its huge profits, the company should find some way to help these people whose lives were changed forever when they worked to clean the beaches of Prince William Sound.

Chapter 6

Gulf War Syndrome

In my book *Gulf War Syndrome: Legacy of a Perfect War* and my video *Gulf War Syndrome: Aftermath of a Toxic Battlefield*, I explored the wide range of toxic exposures that Coalition troops faced in the deserts of Iraq and Kuwait. It was not without reason that Jim Tuite, the chief investigator for the Riegle Senate Banking Committee, which held prolonged hearings on Gulf War syndrome, referred to the area as the "most toxic battlefield in history." My book documents in considerable detail the exposures that caused Tuite to use such a strong phrase. For the purposes of this chapter, however, I shall concentrate on three exposures particularly relevant to the development of chemical sensitivity among a large number of the veterans of the 1991 Gulf War:

- Exposure to nerve agents like sarin
- The pyridostigmine bromide pills taken by large numbers of Coalition troops
- The oil well fires

Exposure to Nerve Agents

One of the greatest dangers facing Coalition forces in the Persian Gulf was the large stocks of nerve agents that Saddam Hussein possessed. As Coalition forces were assembling in Saudi Arabia in late 1990 in response to Iraq's invasion of Kuwait on August 2, 1990, the problem of defending their troops against chemical and biological attacks was uppermost in the minds of Coalition commanders. Intelligence sources had identified twenty-eight chemical weapons factories where deadly nerve agents like sarin, tabun, and VX were being produced.[1] One of the main areas attacked by Coalition bombers when the air war began

---

[1] Jim Tuite, Principal Investigator for the Riegle Committee, footage from the Alison Johnson/Richard Startzman documentary *Gulf War Syndrome: Aftermath of a Toxic Battlefield*.

on January 17, 1991, was a huge complex in the desert located sixty-five miles northwest of Baghdad in an area called Muthanna. The Riegle Committee report noted that according to UN inspectors who visited the site after the war, Muthanna had the capability of producing two tons of sarin and five tons of mustard gas a day.[2] Despite extensive bombing of the site, UN inspectors found at Muthanna after the war seventy-five tons of the nerve agent sarin, twenty-eight SCUD warheads loaded with sarin, and thousands of rockets and bombs loaded with nerve agents.[3]

According to the Riegle Report, "Coalition bombing against these facilities involved hundreds—if not thousands—of tons of bulk chemical nerve agents, mustard gas."[4] In a front-page story on August 14, 1997, *U.S.A. Today* reported:

The Lawrence Livermore National Laboratory had in a 1990 study informed the U.S. Air Force—three months before the Gulf War began—that bombing of Iraqi chemical weapons manufacturing facilities would release deadly nerve agents over U.S. troops who were massing several hundred miles to the south.

The choice for Coalition commanders was indeed difficult. They could either risk having our forces on the receiving end of full-strength attacks with nerve agents if they left the chemical factories and depots in place, or they could take the chance that when they bombed the factories the low levels of nerve agents that might drift over the troops would not be strong enough to cause serious injury to large numbers of soldiers. Few would deny that our commanders made the right decision when they decided the risk of leaving Saddam Hussein's chemical weapons in place was too great to bear.

---

[2] "U.S. Chemical and Biological Warfare-Related Dual Use Exports to Iraq and Their Possible Impact on the Health Consequences of the Persian Gulf War," Senate Committee on Banking, Housing, and Urban Affairs, chaired by Senator Donald W. Riegle, Jr. (D-MI), May 25, 1994, p. 22.

[3] Riegle Report, p. 22.

[4] Riegle Report, p. 24.

On January 17 the air war began, and during the next few weeks Coalition bombers flew hundreds of sorties, attacking all the major Iraqi facilities where chemical or biological weapons were manufactured or stored. From this point on, there would be continuing controversy over the extent to which low levels of chemical agents may have drifted over the troops massing to the south for an eventual ground war.

On January 19, 1991, two days after the air war had begun and the Coalition had started bombing Iraq's chemical weapons facilities, Czech units detected mustard gas and sarin in an area close to the Kuwaiti border. That same day French chemical units also detected low levels of nerve agent in the same general region, about nineteen miles from King Khalid Military City, the huge base in northern Saudi Arabia used as a staging area. It was not until August 1996, however, that the Defense Department at last announced that five years earlier both the French and the Czech chemical troops had detected nerve agents (*New York Times*, October 19, 1996, p. 10).

A Gulf War veteran who spoke on a confidential basis to the staff of Senator Riegle's committee reported that on one occasion between January 20 and February 1, "he was located about 40 miles east of King Khalid Military City (KKMC), when at one position, every M-8 alarm [a chemical agent detection alarm] went off—over 30 at once. . . . The NBC [nuclear/biological/chemical] NCO radioed in that a nerve agent plant had been bombed about 150 miles away. The source recalled that they were told to take no action and they did not."[5]

Sgt. Brian Martin, who served in the 37th Airborne Combat Engineer Battalion, was stationed only six miles from the Iraqi border in late January. He noted in his journal during this period that what were called "false alarms" were going off very frequently. The troops were first told that the alarms were caused by vapors arising from the sand. Eventually when this explanation failed to satisfy anyone, "Martin said he was informed by both his battalion commander and the battalion NBC NCO that the alarms were sounding because of 'minute' quantities of nerve

---

[5] Riegle Report, pp. 97-98.

agent in the air, released by the Coalition bombing of Iraqi chemical weapons facilities. The troops were assured that there was no danger."[6]

These possible exposures to sarin nerve agent and mustard gas were never taken seriously by the Department of Defense, which throughout the decade of the nineties continually minimized the possibility that toxic exposures in the Gulf War had led to long-term illness for Gulf veterans. This attempted DOD coverup was, however, circumvented by Jim Tuite, who stated in his testimony before the Shays Human Resources Subcommittee:

> Using available visible and infrared meteorological satellite imagery from NOAA [National Oceanic and Atmospheric Administration] . . . I have been able to determine that a thermal plume rose into the atmosphere over the largest Iraqi chemical warfare agent research, production, and storage facility at Muthanna after Coalition aircraft and missile bombardment.
>
> Seventeen metric tons of sarin were reportedly destroyed during these attacks, which began on January 17, 1991. These thermal and visual plumes extended [southerly] directly toward the areas where those same chemical warfare agents were detected and confirmed by Czechoslovak chemical specialists. Hundreds of thousands of U.S. servicemen and women were in the area where these detections occurred, assembling for the upcoming ground invasion of Iraq and the liberation of Kuwait.[7]

Once Jim Tuite realized why the chemical detection alarms had sounded so frequently once the Coalition bombing began, he began to focus his attention on the Pentagon's insistence that the alarms had all gone off because of malfunctioning:

> During the congressional investigation into this issue, we found that logs had been kept of chemical detections and chemical

---

[6] Riegle Report, pp. 96-97.

[7] Second Report, "Gulf War Illnesses," by the House Committee on Government Reform and Oversight, Subcommittee on Human Resources, chaired by Congressman Christopher Shays (R-CT), November 7, 1997, p. 24.

activity in the Gulf. We requested these logs, and we were told by the Pentagon in writing that these logs did not exist. Later we found out that in fact these logs did exist. They existed in two secure locations—one in Maryland and one in Florida—and they disappeared from these locations about the time we requested them. These are secure locations intended for security of classified information, and at the time these logs were classified secret. These are secret documents that disappeared from two separate locations simultaneously at the same time that Congress showed an interest in this issue.

> *Gulf War Syndrome: Aftermath of a Toxic Battlefield*
> (hereafter GWS video)

*   *   *   *   *

Khamisiyah

After the ground war ended on February 28, 1991, U.S. commanders decided to blow up the Iraqi ammunition dumps that were scattered across southern Iraq. One of the largest was the vast Khamisiyah complex consisting of about a hundred bunkers in which were stored rockets and other weapons containing sarin nerve agent and cyclosarin. While army intelligence units were aware that deadly nerve agents were stored at Khamisiyah, this information never reached the two engineering units from the 82nd Airborne Division who were assigned to blow up the bunkers at Khamisiyah.

On March 4, 1991, the army engineering units destroyed thirty-seven bunkers in the main area at Khamisiyah; a few days later, on March 9, soldiers investigating the surrounding area discovered large quantities of rockets in an area called the "pit." Because they were running out of some demolition supplies, the plan was not to totally destroy the rockets but to render them inoperable by breaking them apart. If the soldiers had realized that the rockets contained nerve agents, they would have known that it was essential to set large enough explosive charges to burn up the rockets and the chemicals they contained. As it was, they simply set off explosions on March 9 and 10 that broke open the weapons, enabling the nerve agents they contained to escape into the atmosphere or drain into the sand.[8]

After setting the charges, the U.S. troops withdrew to an area about twelve miles away from Khamisiyah. One of the soldiers who helped blow up Khamisiyah was Sgt. Brian Martin, who later described in testimony to the Shays Committee the health problems he had developed after Khamisiyah, which included chemical sensitivity:

> Since Khamisiyah, I suffer from . . . blood in vomit and stools, blurred vision, shaking and trembling . . . muscles weakening . . . chest pounding like my heart was going to explode. . . . I suffer from excruciatingly painful headaches, memory loss, and severe diarrhea . . . mood swings . . . I violently vomit if I smell perfumes, vapors or chemicals. I get lost and forget where I am sometimes. I am an ex-paratrooper who needs a cane and wheelchair to get around. My joints . . . swell, burn and hurt.[9]

Information about what kind of weapons had actually been at Khamisiyah eventually came from UNSCOM, the United Nations Special Commission. According to the Riegle Report: "At the first inspection in October of 1991, UNSCOM found rockets at the Khamisiyah pit and determined that they contained a mixture of sarin and cyclosarin. The rockets that they found included many that were damaged and leaking. UNSCOM also succeeded in finding Iraqi records indicating that approximately 60 tons of sarin and cyclosarin had been placed in 8,000 122mm rockets and over 2,000 of these rockets had ended up at Khamisiyah, half in the main area and half in the pit.

Jim Tuite is highly critical of the DOD's attitude toward the Khamisiyah affair:

---

[8] "Report of the Special Investigation Unit on Gulf War Illnesses," Senate Committee on Veterans' Affairs, chaired by Senator Arlen Specter (R-PA), 1998, p. 24.

[9] Shays Report, p. 11.

Khyamisiyah is only one of hundreds of munition sites and depots that we destroyed after the war whose contents we never inventoried and we destroyed as though there were no risk to troops in the surrounding area. We don't know what was in these bunkers. We didn't know, according to the DOD, what was in Khamisiyah at the time, even though evidence developed afterwards suggest the contrary. But bunker after bunker after bunker was destroyed without any inventory of the contents, without any knowledge of what was being blown up, without any effort to protect the troops in the area to the fallout that may have occurred from these detonations.

When we were conducting the Senate Banking Committee investigation and we first raised this inquiry, we were told by the Pentagon that the fallout couldn't have reached the troops because the wind was blowing in the wrong direction, but we looked at the satellite images and the plumes. The smoke plumes from all the bombing and from the oil well fires that were going on at the same time suggested that the wind was blowing towards the troops. The Pentagon insisted that no chemical agent exposure occurred. In 1996, they admitted, well, maybe at Khamisiyah 185 soldiers may have been exposed, then a few months later, well maybe 400 had been exposed. Then it was 5000, then it was 20,000, then 100,000, then 120,000.

Gulf War Syndrome: Legacy of a Perfect War, pp. 42-43

In 1997 the Pentagon sent letters to almost 98,000 veterans, informing them that computer modeling studies indicated that they might have been exposed to sarin or cyclosarin when Khamisiyah was blown up. Computer models had indicated that the plumes resulting from the explosions could have carried as far as 300 miles to the south and extended over areas where almost 100,000 troops were stationed. [10]

*   *   *   *   *

---

[10] Shays Report, p. 23.

Pyridostigmine Bromide Pills

The U.S. troops called them PB pills, and the British and Australians
called them NAPPs. These tablets contained a drug called pyridostigmine bromide that was given to approximately 250,000 U.S. troops
during Desert Storm in an attempt to protect them against Iraqi use of
nerve agents, or chemical warfare. Was the treatment worse than the
risk of death or extreme disability that would have resulted from an
Iraqi attack with nerve gas? That is one of the lingering issues as
researchers seek for answers to the question of what has caused debilitating illness in so many who served in the Gulf War. These reports come
from veterans who served in the Gulf War:

> The night that the ground war started everyone had to take their
> PB pills. I actually saw one female throwing up from them. I had
> taken about eight. I was so sick at my stomach I quit taking them,
> and I was told by other soldiers they threw theirs away. I'm glad
> I didn't take anymore than I did.
>
> Sfc. Terry Dillhyon, GWS video

> The pills made me feel really strange . . . made my heart race,
> just kind of almost an out-of-body experience. Although I was
> still able to function, things were altered around me, time, space.
> I was more than happy to discontinue taking the things.
>
> S.Sgt. Bob Jones, GWS video

> When I took the PB pills, I was ordered to take them. I did not
> receive nothing about what they would do to you, and they watch
> you take them right in front of you. Basically, what happened
> was, my body just heated up. I seen other personnel in my
> battalion, different reactions of people throwing up, running
> around. Different reactions of different people. Personally,
> myself, I just felt like a big flame, a fire; it was unbelievable.
>
> Sp4c. Bobby Lawson, GWS video

> I had suffered very much with migraine as a teenager, but I
> hadn't suffered for some years. And within, I don't know, maybe
> 48 hours of taking the NAPPs tablets, the PB tablets, I got my

migraines back. And I was aware of stomach dysfunction, I felt nauseous and had more trouble with diarrhea.
                    Sgt. Anne Selby, British veteran, GWS video

The day before the air war, I believe, I would need to check on those dates for sure, but sometime in that time frame we were instructed to take PB pills. We were in fact instructed to go down the line and ensure all our troops actually took the PB pills and swallowed them. Shortly after that, an interesting story, we had a gentleman from our battalion headquarters who went into cardiac arrest, almost within a few hours of taking the first pills. Myself and a reservist who was a physician's assistant from Duke actually started CPR on this individual three times. We went with him all the way to the medivac hospital. They started CPR on him there several times and brought him back, and the interesting part is that after all of that his medical records now show that he had just a pulled muscle in his chest.
                    Sgt. Mike Ange, GWS video footage

Major Doug Rokke, former director of the U.S. Army Depleted Uranium Assessment Project, described PB pills in this way:

The simplest way to understand pyridostigmine bromide, the little white tablets that came in a blister pack, is that they are a carbamate-based pesticide. If you want to think about this, what they did is they went and got you a whole bunch of gumdrops and sprayed them with pesticide and said, "Eat them." Over 50 percent of the people who took the pyridostigmine bromide had immediate pesticide-related health effects. That was expected, that's what's in the physician's desk reference, and what's always been known. You can't eat pesticides and have a good day.
                    Gulf War Syndrome: Legacy of a Perfect War, p. 55

Despite the fact that PB is a highly toxic substance, it has a track record of use over a few decades to treat myasthenia gravis patients. This previous use of PB is discussed in a detailed report on pyridostigmine bromide compiled by the RAND Corporation, which was asked by the DOD to survey existing research on PB. The author of this report, Beatrice Golomb, M.D., is a physician who also has a Ph.D. in biology with a specialization in neurobiology. She is a staff physician at the San Diego VA Medical Center and an assistant professor of medicine at the University of California at San Diego.

One of the many issues that Dr. Golomb investigated in her review of the literature on pyridostigmine bromide was the use of PB to treat myasthenia gravis, a condition in which patients experience increasing weakness in their voluntary muscles because they do not have enough receptors for a neurotransmitter called acetylcholine (ACh) at their neuro-muscular junctions. (ACh acts through ACh receptors on the cell receiving the signal.) The FDA has approved and licensed pyridostigmine bromide for treatment of myasthenia gravis because PB ties up an enzyme called acetylcholinesterase (AChE) that breaks down ACh after it has served its purpose. AChE helps increase the amount of ACh in these myasthenia gravis patients, so that the reduced number of ACh receptor cells will have a better chance of receiving the nerve signal properly.

As Dr. Golomb so cogently notes, however, although myasthenia gravis patients tolerate dosage levels of PB that are considerably higher than those given to our troops, PB moves these patients toward a normal state, while PB given to a healthy person will move that person away from a normal state. "One analogy is the difference between how insulin affects diabetics and those not suffering from the condition. A severe diabetic may tolerate or require 60 units of insulin or more each day to bring his or her blood sugar *toward* normal. Yet far smaller doses may induce hypoglycemic coma or even death in a nondiabetic subject."[11]

There was a reason, however, why Coalition commanders turned to the toxic PB pills to protect their troops. To follow their logic, one must first understand how nerve agents work to wreak havoc in the bodies of humans and other animals and produce almost certain death if no antidote is available. They damage living organisms by interfering with one of the most basic physiological systems of the body—the

---

[11] RAND Corporation, "A Review of the Scientific Literature As It Pertains to Gulf War Illnesses," vol. 2, " Pyridostigmine Bromide," by Beatrice Golomb, chap. 3, p. 8.

cholinergic system that enables nerve cells to send messages to muscle cells or other nerve cells.

The neurotransmitter called acetylcholine (ACh) is essential for the control of muscles, both voluntary and involuntary, as well as for brain function. A nerve cell uses acetylcholine to send a signal, for example, to a muscle cell to cause contraction or relaxation of the muscle. Normally, an enzyme called acetylcholinesterase (AChE) breaks down the ACh after it has served its purpose. Nerve agents act by binding to AChE, preventing it from breaking down ACh. The result is a buildup of ACh at the junction between the nerve cell and the cell to which it is sending a signal. This buildup of ACh at these crucial junctions where messages are passed to other nerve cells or muscle cells that initiate a wide range of cellular activity can lead to malfunction throughout the body.

As the RAND report notes, a buildup of ACh can cause GI symptoms like cramping, nausea, diarrhea, and vomiting; tearing of the eyes; runny nose; bronchospasm; frequent urination; and bladder or bowel incontinence. The report also raises the question of whether the PB pills the soldiers took in the Gulf could have caused an ongoing dysregulation in the cholinergic system.

Sgt. Roy Twymon, who has suffered from migraines, joint pains, rashes, lesions on his legs, and fatigue since the war, has described the devastating effect that incontinence problems have had upon his life:

> From the time we was given the PB pill, we was told to continue to take them. We kept on taking them, and we kept on taking them till after the war. And I noticed then that I started having diarrhea, my bowel was a different color, I had to run to the outdoor toilet because sometime, you know, it be that severe, the diarrhea does, you know. I started noticing . . . I couldn't hold my bladder.
>
> And this kept on happening, kept on happening, kept on happening while we was over there. Then when we got back, my soldiers started complaining, and they was sent to the hospital, sent to psych, told it was all in their head.
>
> I kept on dealing with it, and one day [after I got back] it really hurt me and struck me. I was coming from fishing with my son, and I wasn't even a block away from the Seven-Eleven in

San Antonio, Texas, and I couldn't even make it to the Seven-Eleven, and I soiled on myself. I knew then there was something terrible wrong with me.

Then as I went on with my bowel and bladder problem, I realized what was going on, and when I ran into some of the individuals that was in my unit, some of the guys, I would pull them aside and ask them if they was having some of the same problems. . . . And all of them that I spoke to said yes, they was having the same problems and some more problems. . . .

They found nerve damage to my internal sphincter muscle. The sphincter muscle is the one that helps hold your bowel. So when you have to go to the bathroom or get the urge to go, you have to be whupped in the bathroom, or you'd best be running, or you just go on yourself. And I know that a forty-four-year-old, I'm forty-four-years-old now, and I know there's forty-four-year-old men that haven't been to the Gulf War don't have this problem. So, you know, it started when I came back, and I know it happened over there because there's too many of us having the same problem. . . .   I miss a lot of events with my kids, you know, their activities. My son plays college football. Could you imagine me going to a college football game, eighty, ninety thousand people trying to get into the same restroom with you? No, I'd soil on myself, so all of these activities and things that my kids have been into since I've been back and the things that I've missed, no one can give that back to me, no one.

GWS video

As Sgt. Twymon's statement about other soldiers he served with having similar incontinence problems indicates, incontinence among the Gulf veterans is probably more widespread than is realized because people find it extremely embarrassing to admit that they have this symptom. Sgt. Bob Jones, a former paratrooper who served in an artillery unit in Desert Storm, has admitted that he shares this difficulty:

Things just got to the point where I had diarrhea on myself at work a couple of times, and I said, enough is enough, I need to get help. It's real embarrassing to be standing around all your men and all of a sudden you can't even make it to the bathroom on time.

GWS video

But despite all the problems that usage of PB may have caused, there were compelling reasons for the Pentagon to decide that it was the lesser of evils when the alternative was death or severe injury from nerve agents. The problem is not so much that the decision was made to order our troops to take PB but that the DOD and VA do not seem to be willing to admit that PB could be a large factor in the present debilitating health problems that the Gulf veterans are experiencing and to take responsibility for their care or support in the cases of those who are unable to work.

This question of the accumulation of PB in the body becomes even more serious if we consider the research of Mohamed Abou-Donia, Ph.D., a professor of pharmacology at Duke University Medical School. Dr. Abou-Donia has shown that when PB is given to rodents in combination with other chemicals encountered during the Gulf War, the blood brain barrier breaks down, allowing toxic substances and pathogens in the bloodstream to enter the brain.[12]

*   *   *   *   *

The Oil Well Fires

As the Iraqi forces retreated from Kuwait at the end of the war, they set huge numbers of oil wells on fire in what can only be viewed as the ultimate in a scorched earth tactic. A small number of oil wells were also ignited by Coalition bombing of nearby targets. The fires peaked as the ground war began on February 24, and by late February, over 600 oil wells were ablaze and 85 percent of Kuwait's oil production facilities had been damaged. A DOD report titled *Oil Well Fires* notes:

---

[12] *Gulf War Syndrome: Legacy of a Perfect War*, by Alison Johnson, 2001, pp. 66-68.

The damaged well heads released approximately 4-6 million barrels of crude oil and 70-100 million cubic meters of natural gas per day. . . .

The burning wells created a huge, widely dispersed smoke plume that degraded the region's air quality and released various potentially hazardous gases, including sulfur dioxide (SO_2), carbon monoxide (CO), hydrogen sulfide (H_2S), carbon dioxide (CO_2) and nitrogen oxides (NO_x), and particulate matter (soot) that potentially contained partially burned hydrocarbons and metals. If sufficiently concentrated, both gases and particulate matter potentially can impair health in exposed populations.[13]

The DOD also commissioned a RAND report titled *Oil Well Fires*. The report's author, Dalia M. Spektor, notes that "SO_2 is an upper-airway irritant that can stimulate bronchoconstriction and mucus secretion. Animal studies indicate that relatively low concentration exposures of SO_2 (0.1 to 20 ppm) for long periods have marked effects consistent with bronchitis.[14]

In a *Science* magazine article published May 15, 1992, researchers Peter V. Hobbs and Lawrence F. Radke state: "Close to the fires the smoke rained oil drops. . . . This oil, together with soot fallout, coated large areas of the desert with a black, tar-like covering. Oil spewing out from uncapped wells formed large pools of oil on the desert, some of which were alight." This immense conflagration resembled nothing so much as a scene from hell, and our soldiers who were caught in it retain indelible memories of the event, as S.Sgt. Bob Jones recounted in my GWS book:

After the cease-fire, we ended up spending 45 days in the Rhumali oil fields in the midst of the burning oil wells. It was just incredible, something surreal, like being in another world. We saw no sunlight for almost all that time because the sun was completely blackened out by the smoke and soot. The vapors of

---

[13] DOD Report, *Oil Well Fires,* chap. 3, p. 1.

[14] Ibid., chap. 3, p. 11.

burning fuel were terrible—it was like breathing diesel exhaust constantly. It became so bad at times that I put on my protective mask to try to filter out some clean air. I had severe headaches and was nauseous from the fumes. There were particles falling out of the sky on top of us, and we had a black film and soot on our skin. It was just unbelievable to be sitting in something like that. We kept wondering why they didn't move us away from this area where we were continuously breathing in all this crap.

Gulf War Syndrome, pp. 192-93

I was in Kuwait, and we had sixty oil wells burning where I was. A lot of people got sick, they had asthma attacks. People that had never had asthma before had asthma during Kuwait. We were coughing up until we got back to Germany. I still coughed up and it was black and for six months afterwards, I was still coughing up black.

Sgt. Sherrie McGahee, GWS video footage

I have obstructive pulmonary disease, which I attribute to the smoke in Kuwait City. Where I was stationed, close to Camp Freedom in Kuwait City, you couldn't tell night from day. If you saw a globe in the sky, you didn't know whether it was the moon or the sun. My skin was so black you couldn't tell my skin from my black watch band. When you spit, it looked like oil, when you blew your nose, it looked like axle grease. That's the kind of pollution I'm talking about. The doctor who diagnosed me said, "Well, you've got this obstructive pulmonary disease because you smoke cigarettes." And I said, "No, a cigarette has never touched my lips in my entire life, unless you want to count what happened to me in Kuwait, which is probably the equivalent to a thousand packs of cigarettes a day."

It was seventeen days before we had enough water that any of us could take a shower. We took the shower, in a tent of course, closed in. We got clean until we opened the tent door and put on our dirty, oil-soaked clothing because we didn't have enough water for laundry.

Col. Herbert Smith, *Gulf War Syndrome*, p. 151

At one point during the war, we were staying near the oil wells and your uniform would be completely covered with black, like soot all over you. Your arms were exposed, your food, everything, your water where you took showers. It was constantly dark, there was no such thing as daylight.

Sp4c. Bobby Lawson, GWS video footage

My breathing was not good. My breathing felt very much as though I was trying to take in glue instead of air. It was not pleasant. And that continued until after we came back to the UK. . . . and then I became very ill in the first week I started university, which would be in September of 1991. And it progressed into pneumonia, but I didn't realize it was pneumonia at first. . . .

They gave me all of these antibiotics. They just tried me on one after another. Nothing worked, and then finally it seemed to settle down for a little while. Then at Christmas of that year I became ill again, and this time I got pneumonia very badly. It was what my doctor called atypical pneumonia. And because I'd had pneumonia twice within the space of three months, they decided to put me in hospital to find out what was going on. And when they actually looked at my lungs, they said that there was a lot of oily debris in my lungs. . . . I didn't connect for some reason the oily debris bit and the oil well fires bit. I didn't connect it immediately. And they asked me, "Have you been in a house fire?" and I said no. And they said, "Well, we can't understand why your lungs are in such bad shape."

By the time I returned for a review appointment in two weeks I had actually made the connection. I went back to the doctor, and I said, "Look, would oil wells have done it, burning oil wells?" And he looked at me and he said yes. He said, "When were you with burning oil? You don't work in the oil industry, do you?" I said, "No, but I was a soldier out in the Gulf." And he said, "Ah, yes. because the fumes from burning oil wells are both toxic and carcinogenic. They set fire to something they call the signature, which is highly toxic."

The official diagnosis for my lung problems and my breathing difficulties is bronchiectasis, which is scarring of the tissue of the surface of the lung. And they just put me on inhalers and various things, and really I've been that way ever since because there's really nothing they can do. The lungs will only heal themselves to a certain extent. They won't completely heal, so I'm stuck with the problem until I die. . . .

I can't walk for long distances without my lungs filling up with fluid. Your lungs try to protect you by producing more fluid, so basically what happens is that I start choking, coughing on the fluid after I've walked for a little while. Running is out of the question. . . .

I can't go back to doing what I originally did–I was a singer, a stage performer. Even though I can still sing, there is no way I've got the lung capacity now to carry x-amount of tunes for x-amount of hours a night. So there's no way I can go back to my former profession I had before I joined the Army . . .

A media person did ask me the other day if there was any important statement that I would care to make about my experience in the Gulf, and basically I laughed and said, "Well, apart from the fact that it's absolutely destroyed my life, I'm not sure what else to say."

Sgt. Anne Selby, *Gulf War Syndrome*, pp. 186-88

Given the reports from those unfortunate enough to have been forced to spend weeks by the burning oil wells, it seems hard to believe that the risk to health from this exposure would not have been great. Nevertheless, the 1998 RAND report entitled *Oil Well Fires*, which was commissioned by the Department of Defense, dismisses the possibility of any health risks from exposure to these fires. The summary states: "The level of pollutants measured in the Gulf were much lower than those that are known to cause short- or long-term health effects." The problem is that the RAND Corporation and other groups evaluating the relationship of Gulf War syndrome to the oil well fires all relied upon data collected starting in May 1991, when the very strong Shamal winds had started to blow in the Persian Gulf. By the time the Army started measuring the pollution, a large percentage of our forces had already left the Gulf, undoubtedly carrying away with them soot particles in their lungs and toxic petroleum chemicals in their fatty tissue. S.Sgt. Fred Willoughby, who died in 2004, reports: "When I got home, there was a lot of months that I would have heavy sweating and the bed sheets and pillow cases on my side of the bed were black from all the stuff coming out of my skin."[15]

A very different view from that expressed in the RAND report is found in the paper entitled *Oil Fires, Petroleum and Gulf War Illness*, which was written by Craig Stead, a chemical engineer and expert on health effects related to exposure to petroleum. Stead submitted his paper to the 1999 CDC Conference on the Health Impact of Chemical Exposures During the Gulf War. In testimony to the Shays subcommittee, Stead stated:

> In 1994, the Army issued the final Kuwait Oil Fire Health Risk Assessment. The Assessment used Gulf air pollution data gathered in May through November 1991. Air pollution from the oil field fires during this time was much less than during the Gulf War for the following reasons: The months of May through November [when the study was done] have the Shamal winds blowing from the northwest causing the smoke plume from the oil field fires to disperse widely and ascend to great heights. During the Gulf War (February and March) low wind speeds and air inversions were common. Under these conditions the smoke plume was on the ground, creating high localized levels of air pollution to which the troops were exposed.[16]

Stead focused not only on the inversion episodes but also on the soldiers' exposure to soot and oil rain. The oil rain resulted because in many cases a jet of unburned oil shot up through the flames, and the oil that was thus dispersed throughout the atmosphere eventually fell to earth as an oil rain, coating the uniforms and any exposed skin of the soldiers in the area. Stead quotes from an early version of the DOD oil well fire report an especially horrific account of this toxic rain:

> [We] traveled the "coastal highway," from Kuwait City down to Saudi Arabia . . . and the petroleum-thickened air was so impregnated that we choked on oil while breathing through our

---

[15] Alison Johnson, *Gulf War Syndrome: Legacy of a Perfect War*, p. 213.

[16] Shays Report, p. 32.

doubled-up scarves. . . . We were forced to stop and clear the
raw petroleum off vehicle windshields and our goggles constantly. At [times] on the highway the . . . air was so thick our
vehicle headlights could not penetrate the air further than 10-15
feet, and Marine escorts were needed to walk . . . ahead of the
vehicles to keep us on the highway.[17]

It would hardly be unwarranted to suggest that exposures like this would
in all likelihood be a strong contributing factor to Gulf War syndrome.
The DOD report on the oil well fires also refers obliquely to the oil rain:

The most severe exposures to U.S. troops from the oil well fires
occurred when they were in proximity to the damaged or burning
wells. During these incidences, troops were subjected to short-
term exposures where they were literally drenched in unburned
oil and/or covered with fall-out (i.e., soot, smoke, and other by-
products of combustion) from the oil well fires.[18]

One very important health consequence that government researchers
may be missing is the sensitization to chemicals that seems to have
occurred with so many Gulf soldiers. In my interviews with ill veterans,
almost all of them have mentioned an extreme sensitivity to petroleum
products, a sensitivity that they never had before the war. And this
sensitivity seems to have spread over the years to other chemical
substances:

I had spent eight years in the 82nd Airborne Division as a
paratrooper, so I had had extensive exposure to jet fuel and jet
fumes, and these things had never bothered me. But having spent
forty-five days in the area where the oil wells were burning,
breathing the noxious fumes on a daily basis, now just the smell
of diesel fuel makes me severely nauseated, dizzy, and very sick.
I try to avoid getting behind school buses because diesel exhaust
really bothers me, as do other odors and smells. Perfumes are

---

[17] *Oil Fires, Petroleum and guf War Illness,* Craig Stead, p. 35.

[18] DOD Report, *Oil Well Fires,* chap. 5, p. 3.

also a problem; I don't wear any type of cologne because it
makes me nauseous.

S.Sgt. Bob Jones, *Gulf War Syndrome*, p. 194

Gasoline—that makes me sick at my stomach.

Sgt. Sherrie McGahee, GWS video

I couldn't pump my own gas . . . the gas fumes would make me
vomit. . . . If I breathed automobile fumes, truck fumes, again I'm
nauseous, trying to not vomit.

Col. Herb Smith, GWS video

I have problems breathing on buses because of the diesel fumes
and to some extent with cars because of the petrol fumes. I have
problems using household disinfectants and chemicals because
it causes my airways to close, and it causes me to start choking.

Sgt. Anne Selby, GWS video footage

When my husband first came back from Saudi, to even put gas
in his vehicle, he would throw up. To change oil, his hands, it
looked like little worms would come out on his hands. And they
told him he had an allergic reaction to petroleum products. . . .
Whenever I would use a pine-scented cleaner, when he'd get out
of the truck, he would have to get right back in, he couldn't even
come in the house. He would just start throwing up.

Margaret Wilcoxen, GWS video

The biggest thing is the sensitivity to stuff. You used to go out
all the time and paint your house and use the thinners and stuff,
and now you've got to avoid the use of the thinners. When you
pump your own gas, like myself, I've got to turn away so I don't
breathe the fumes. The chemical sensitivity is becoming just
unreal, and you notice it now. Before, when you would pump
gas, you used to stand there and smell the fumes, you know,
great, this stuff don't bother me. And now you've got to try to
hide and pump at the same time.

Sgt. Tim Smith, GWS video

My problems with chemical sensitivity began right after the Gulf
War. I still cannot pump gas or diesel fuel; my wife pumps it

while I sit in the car or truck with the windows rolled up. [When I went back to work], I started having problems that I never had before. The automatic air freshener dispenser in our office was making me sick, as were paint and diesel fumes.

Sfc. Terry Dillhyon, GWS video footage

For the veterans suffering from Gulf War syndrome, the chemical sensitivity that they developed in the war is a burden that affects every aspect of their lives, and in particular, their ability to work. Mechanics who have become sensitive to petroleum products can no longer repair cars or other machinery. On our GWS video, Sfc. Terry Dillhyon and Sfc. Roy Twymon both describe perfume exposures that put them in the hospital for a couple of days. Trying to find a job where one can avoid exposure to substances like gasoline, solvents, paint, cleaning products, new carpet, diesel exhaust, perfume, and aftershave lotion quickly becomes an exercise in frustration, as was indicated in Chapter 1. It is only just that the government provide financial assistance to these ill veterans whose lives were changed forever by their heroic service in the Gulf War.

Chapter 7

The World Trade Center Disaster

One could argue that on 9/11 the claim to being the most toxic battle-field in history passed from the deserts of Kuwait and Iraq to the Ground Zero area of Lower Manhattan. While the Twin Towers crumbled in less than a hour, the struggle in the early hours and days to find survivors and the ensuing months-long cleanup efforts resulted in the exposure of 40,000 city, state, and federal workers, including the particularly heroic First Responders, to a frightening array of toxic substances. And these government workers were not the only ones exposed. Volunteers rushed to the site, and hundreds of thousands of people live and work in Lower Manhattan in the areas contaminated by the smoke and dust that contained asbestos, dioxin, lead, mercury, arsenic, and a host of other dangerous substances. Significant numbers are now suffering a wide array of chronic health problems.

Like so many other health care professionals across the city, and indeed the country, Dr. Stephen Levin, Medical Director of the Mount Sinai Occupational and Environmental Clinic, was appalled in the early days after the attack that people were not being warned how dangerous the Ground Zero site was:

> Well, we were horrified on September 18, 2001, when the head of the EPA, Christine Todd Whitman, got on television and said she was glad to be able to reassure people that the air quality was safe. I remember listening to that and being aghast, just horrified that she could say such a thing. . . . I knew that she didn't have the data to be able to make such a statement, that at that point there was very limited monitoring that had been done.
>
> . . . . .
>
> Initially, there was a strong suspicion that many of us had that this was a decision, this pronouncement about the safety of air quality down there, that was based less on public health and less on monitoring data than a desire to get Lower Manhattan running

economically, get Wall Street going, get the Stock Exchange going. There was a lot of talk about that. It wasn't until later that we had confirmation that, lo and behold, this really was a strong influence on the EPA's pronouncements because it turned out that the Council on Environmental Quality, the president's own sub-cabinet-level group in the White House, had influenced what the EPA was going to say. In fact, the EPA had been preparing to issue a cautionary message saying, "We're not sure what's going on down there but you ought to be careful because this in fact may be a toxic environment." What the Council on Environmental Quality said to the EPA was "Emphasize reassurance, de-emphasize hazard," and so the EPA reversed itself.

Toxic Clouds of 9/11 video

Dr. Levin's fears were well founded, as was established by the research that he later performed as Co-Director of the World Trade Center Medical Monitoring Program. In that program, he and his fellow researchers at Mount Sinai discovered high rates of both upper respiratory and lower respiratory problems among those who had been exposed to the black smoke that shrouded the Ground Zero area and reached as far as Brooklyn:

We did an analysis of about a ten percent sample of our 12,000 examinees, and among them just about half had symptoms involving their lower respiratory system, their chest–shortness of breath, chest tightness, cough, wheezing. And about another half had upper respiratory symptoms–sinusitis, facial pressure, headaches, stuffy nose, post-nasal drip, the kind of classic symptoms of sinusitis.

Toxic Clouds of 9/11 video

The EPA's concerted efforts to downplay the toxic exposures near Ground Zero are documented in detail in an excellent report that can be found on the website of the Sierra Club.[1] As Suzanne Mattei, who was until recently the head of the NYC Sierra Club office, stated on my 9/11 documentary:

---

[1] www.sierraclub/groundzero/report2005.

We would have been better off if EPA had said nothing at all
because if EPA had said nothing at all, people would have used
their common sense. They would have said, "Looks bad. Smells
bad. Probably shouldn't breathe it in." But EPA said, "It's fine.
It's safe. We've tested. Come back." And everybody came back,
and thousands and thousands of people were exposed.

The failure of the EPA to sound the warning about the myriad dangers
lurking in the WTC dust and fumes had long-reaching consequences not
only for those working on the pile and trucking away the debris, but also
for those living or working near Ground Zero. Many workers have
reported that when they objected to being asked to return to workplaces
that were full of dust and smoke, they were told that they had no choice
if they wanted to keep their jobs because Christine Todd Whitman, the
head of the EPA, had announced on September 18, just six days after
9/11, "I am glad to reassure the people of New York and Washington,
D.C., that their air is safe to breathe."

Whitman's reassuring pronouncement laid the groundwork for the
decision that it was safe to reopen Stuyvesant High School a few weeks
after 9/11, even though the school was located immediately adjacent to
the site on the Hudson River where a seemingly endless line of trucks
dumped their loads of WTC debris onto barges that took it over to
Staten Island to be deposited at the Fresh Kills landfill (thus shifting
much of Manhattan's toxic problem to Staten Island). To make matters
worse, the Stuyvesant auditorium had served as a triage center during
the first few weeks after the terrorist attack. The First Responders,
cleanup crews, and search dogs would retreat there to regroup, leaving
the toxic dust that covered the dog's fur and people's clothing on the
carpet and the upholstered auditorium seats. Testing implemented by a
parents' group showed high levels of asbestos in the carpet and lead in
the ventilation system, but the school administrators insisted upon
reopening the school anyway.

The air quality was so bad near Ground Zero during the months
following 9/11 that they were paying people to live there. An article that
appeared in May of 2002 in *Time Out* magazine, a New York City
publication about what to see and do in the city, describes an unusual
plan announced by the Lower Manhattan Development Corporation.
Under this plan, the LMDC offered to subsidize the rent of anyone who
would sign a two-year lease to live in the area near Ground Zero before

June 1, 2003. The money for this expensive program was to come from the state government. Those living in the area closest to the World Trade Center were to receive a subsidy equal to thirty percent of their monthly rent or mortgage, with a cap of $12,000 over a two-year period. And parents who brought children with them into this area where their health might be jeopardized would get an extra one-time payment of $1,500, an incentive that appalled many observers.

Subsidizing people to rent apartments in the area around Ground Zero was particularly dubious when it had been well documented by the Sierra Club and the New York Environmental Law and Justice Project that many of the WTC dust samples contained high levels of asbestos. Exposure to asbestos can decades later cause the development of lung cancer and mesothelioma, cancer of the lining of the lungs. Congressman Jerrold Nadler, who represents the district containing Ground Zero, noted in his 2003 White Paper concerning the toxic legacy of 9/11 that New York City and New York State have implemented policies that may expose them to a myriad of lawsuits as New Yorkers develop serious health problems over the next few decades:

> By providing residents with inappropriate guidance regarding apartment cleaning, the city may amass huge contingent liabilities. Similarly, New York State, by providing incentives for individuals to move into Lower Manhattan (via the Lower Manhattan Development Corporation)–at a time when the area may not be safe–may also be accruing these liabilities.

Congressman Nadler, who received the Earth Day New York/Natural Resources Defense Council's 2003 "Public Official of the Year" award, released a press release expressing his outrage that Christine Todd Whitman had appeared at the event:

> Without a doubt, Administrator Whitman has led an agency that has done more harm to New Yorkers than perhaps all of the previous Administrations combined. For her to come to New York on Earth Day and pretend she is a friend to New York and its environment is a complete sham. . . . Under Administrator Whitman, the EPA bucked its responsibility under Federal law to clean up interior spaces of New York City that were–and continue to be–contaminated with hazardous materials released by the collapse of the World Trade Center. In ten years or so, this City will see an explosion in cases of cancer, mesothelioma, and

other respiratory diseases that will dwarf the problems many New Yorkers already have faced because of contaminated interiors. We will look back at this Earth Day, when she pretends to be helping New Yorkers, and wonder how anyone could perpetrate such a farce.

Some of the best information about what the WTC dust contained was obtained by Dr. Thomas Cahill, a physicist at the University of California at Davis, and his DELTA Group (Detection and Evaluation of Long-range Transport of Aerosols). Working under contract to the U.S. Geological Service, Cahill and his fellow scientists gathered samples of the WTC dust. The results of their study appear on the University of California at Davis website, which quotes Davis as saying:

> Now that we have a model of how the debris pile worked, it gives us a much better idea of what the people working on and near the pile were actually breathing. . . . The debris pile acted like a chemical factory. It cooked together the components of the buildings and their contents, including enormous numbers of computers, and gave off gases of toxic metals, acids and organics for at least six weeks.

The website also reported that Dr. Cahill had said that the toxic nature of the dust indicated that people who worked without respirators at Ground Zero encountered "brutal" conditions, and the situation was only slightly better for those who worked or lived in the immediate neighborhood. Cahill's group, which has studied pollution all across the world, found that the WTC level of pollutants was worse than those they had encountered in China or in the oil well fires in Kuwait during the Gulf War.

Andrew Schneider was the first investigative journalist to bring to the nation's attention the dangerously high alkalinity levels of some of the World Trade Center dust. In his February 9, 2002, article that appeared in the *St. Louis Post-Dispatch*, he released some of the results of Dr. Cahill's study, which showed that a few dust samples had an alkalinity as high as 12, an alkalinity similar to that of drain cleaner, and many other samples had an alkalinity of 11, which is similar to that of ammonia. Reporter Schneider quoted Dr. Robin Herbert, Dr. Levin's co-director of the WTC Medical Monitoring Program, as raising concerns about the possible effects of this high alkalinity:

> What we're finding is incredible irritation to the lungs, throat and nasal passages. Some of the tissue is cherry red, vivid, bright, and we've never seen anything like it before. . . . The high pH in the dust may be part of the answer. If the government had these pH readings of 11 and 12, the public and their physicians should have been told.

On February 11, two days after Schneider's article appeared, a U.S. Senate subcommittee that deals with clean air issues held a special field hearing in Lower Manhattan at which Senators Hillary Clinton and Joe Lieberman were asked to preside because they represent two of the states that lost the most citizens when the Twin Towers collapsed. When Congressman Jerrold Nadler cited at that hearing Dr. Cahill's finding that some of the WTC dust was as caustic as drain cleaner, there was an audible gasp from the stunned audience that had filled the auditorium. In effect, many of the heroic First Responders and cleanup workers had been breathing in dust that was so caustic that it resembled drain cleaner or ammonia once it reached the moist mucus membranes of their nose, throat, and lungs.

Having attended this Senate hearing investigating the toxic exposures related to the collapse of the Twin Towers and the fires that burned at Ground Zero for months, I was eager to read the *New York Times* coverage of this major event. To my great surprise, the *New York Times* did not cover the hearing at all. I had expected at least a half page would be devoted to this major Senate field hearing near Ground Zero, but the *New York Times* didn't even bury the story in a sentence or two deep within the paper. The *Los Angeles Times*, the *Times* of London, *USA Today*, and the *Washington Post* all covered the event, but as far as the *New York Times* was concerned, this Senate hearing on WTC air quality never happened. The newspaper instead conveniently ran on the day after the hearing a full-page story describing the condition of the buildings encircling the gaping hole at Ground Zero, a story that could have been printed at any time. One can only speculate about the reluctance of the decision makers and owners at the *New York Times* to run a story having huge financial implications for insurance companies and the owners of real estate in Lower Manhattan.

The headlines for many of the stories about possible 9/11 health problems that ran in the *New York Times* for months, and indeed over a year, following 9/11 might just as well have all read "Not to Worry." An October 11, 2001, article was titled "Contaminants Below Levels for Long-Term Concerns"; a March 3, 2002, article was titled "With Glee, P.S. 89 Pupils Go 'Home': Ground Zero"; and a December 24, 2002, article was titled "9/11 Dust Seen as Less Toxic Than Feared." At last another *New York Times* reporter, Anthony DePalma, published several articles that took the WTC toxic risk seriously. In a May 13, 2006, article that was titled "Tracing Lung Ailments That Rose With 9/11 Dust," DePalma wrote:

> But there are already clear signs that the dust, smoke and ash that responders breathed in have led to an increase in diseases that scar the lungs and reduce their capacity to take in and let out air.
>
> The Fire Department tracked a startling increase in cases of a particular lung scarring disease, known as sarcoidosis, among firefighters, which rose to five times the expected rate in the two years after Sept. 11.

An article that appeared in the *New York Daily News* on July 24, 2006, noted other problems for firefighters: "Most stunningly, FDNY doctors calculated that the average lung capacity of Ground Zero firefighters and EMS [Emergency Medical Services] workers had decreased by the equivalent of 12 years of aging."

The media tends to engage in intense coverage of the immediate aftermath of sensational events like the Sago mine disaster, the *Exxon Valdez* oil spill, or the destruction of the World Trade Center. This can have negative consequences, a major one being that the media focus tends to produce a frenzied rush to take action as quickly as possible when much might be gained by a more measured analysis of the situation before monumental efforts to deal with the damage are launched. In the recent Utah mine disaster, the heavy media coverage may have been in part responsible for the unwise decision to send rescue workers into a dangerous situation in which three of them lost their lives. In

Chapter 5, we saw that intense media coverage pushed Exxon to take actions in Alaska that in retrospect can be considered debatable.

After the first few days of a feverish search for 9/11 survivors, there was a switch in media focus to the plight of families who wanted to recover at least some remains of their missing loved ones, who were now presumed dead. "Give the families something to bury" was a recurrent phrase in the media. This media mantra served to encourage cleanup crews to work under conditions such that every breath they drew contained toxic dust, and some of that dust was as caustic as drain cleaner. The sad irony of the 9/11 recovery efforts is that the search through the toxic debris for body parts of the terrorists' victims almost certainly will be seen as the years pass to have condemned large numbers of people to an early death or a lifetime of debilitating illness.

When I first showed my *Toxic Clouds of 9/11* documentary in New York City, a Japanese television crew filmed that screening and the panel discussion that followed. It was clear that, like me, they saw the likely parallel to Hiroshima and Nagasaki: not only a large number of initial deaths but many more to follow over the ensuing decades.

Attorney David Worby is now directing a major lawsuit whose plaintiffs include over ten thousand federal, state, or city employees who worked at Ground Zero and are now chronically ill, many of them unable to work. There remains, however, one largely unheralded group that was key to cleaning up the dust-filled office and apartment buildings in order to get the stock market and America's financial hub running again. Contractors hastily gathered up thousands of day laborers–some off street corners–to perform this crucial work. Many were immigrants, and some were undocumented. In most cases, they were not given masks. Some workers who brought along their own dust masks were told not to wear them because it would make their fellow workers nervous about the working conditions.

In the summer of 2006, a social worker who helps immigrant families related to me her concerns about the health of the children whom many of these workers had taken to work with them. All day long these children had sat in debris-filled rooms, breathing in the clouds of toxic dust that their parents were sweeping up or vacuuming. Lead, a toxin that is particularly dangerous for children, was one of the many substances in the dust. One significant lead source was the tens of thousands of computers that were burned or pulverized when the Twin

Towers collapsed and burned. In November 2001, the National Institute of Environmental Health Sciences stated, "Computer monitors may contain as much as four pounds of lead each" and also noted, "it was common practice at the time of the construction of the buildings to use lead-based paint to rustproof steel beams."[2] The social worker said that many of these children who watched their parents clean the buildings are now sick, but their parents have nowhere to turn for medical care because they are undocumented workers.

Alex Sanchez, his mother Iris Romero, and his friend Manuel Checo, immigrants from the Dominican Republic who are now U.S. citizens, worked long hours in the buildings around Ground Zero, removing dust that was sometimes several inches high. They worked twelve-hour shifts, seven days a week. The men worked for six months; Iris for three months. One difficult job that Alex and Manuel were assigned was to remove the dust from the vents and duct work of the HVAC systems in these offices and apartments. One man would stand at one end of a duct with a blower, while the other would stand at the other end with a vacuum on his shoulder to pick up the dust being blown through the duct. Obviously, a lot of the dust was entering not only the vacuum cleaner but also the lungs of the man holding the vacuum.

When we filmed Alex, then thirty-nine, his mother Iris, his five-year-old son Jack, and his friend Manuel for *The Toxic Clouds of 9/11*, Alex described their difficult situation in poignant terms:

> We are extremely sick. Most of our symptoms are chronic. Manuel and myself are developing nodules in our lungs. We suffer from post-traumatic stress disorder and gastrointestinal reflux. We get devastating pain in our stomach. I need to take eighteen medications on a daily basis. I'm suffering from joint pains. First there was the hip pain. . . . My knees [are] swollen right this minute, and I'm in extreme pain.
>
> I feel extremely, how can I say this, scared and at times panicky. My mother is helping me raise my son and not only because of that, this is my mother. I'm her only child, and when

---

[2] "NIEHS Responds to World Trade Center Attacks," *Environmental Health Perspectives* 109, no. 11 (November 2001): A535.

I see my mother drain blood from her nose like it's a faucet, it's extremely scary. And when I see my mother that has been hospitalized three times already and hooked up to machines, it's not a pretty sight.

It took me three years to get partially compensated. My mother has not been compensated yet. Frustration sets in immediately when you are in pain and also you're having the bill collector at your door knocking. It's like adding insult to injury. Like I said, we owe this man [Manuel Checo] big time. He carried my family financially and gave us moral support. There came times where I just wanted to end it all, and I don't feel ashamed of saying this because the walls were closing in on me. But I would look at my son on a daily basis, and that has given me the fight to continue the struggle, to continue to bring awareness, to go to Capitol Hill, to speak to members of Congress.

Before 9/11, I was earning roughly $700 a week. Today I've been partially compensated by workers' comp, and the insurance is paying me $243 a week. Manuel was earning $131 from workers' compensation. Then Manuel lived out of his car because he lost his apartment and couldn't pay his bills. Go figure. If you're earning $700 a week, and now you're given $131 from the workers' compensation board, you can only expect havoc.

It's only been, what, five years now, and every day goes by we feel worse and worse, and we're cranky and we're anxious and we're mad and we cry, we're depressed. But it's because we see ourselves deteriorating.

Dr. Stephen Levin has been outraged by the way the workers' compensation system has treated the people who worked in one way or another to clean up the Ground Zero area:

We thought that in the light of what the World Trade Center events indicated and the remarkable heroism that so many of these volunteers and workers showed that the workers' compensation insurance companies in New York State would behave differently, that they would be more lenient, less challenging, less willing to fight tooth and nail over each case. But in fact that turned out not to be the situation. If anything, the rates of contra-version, and that's a term that means fighting a case, denying a case, were even higher for World Trade Center responders than they are usually for occupational disease cases. And that's unconscionable.

Toxic Clouds of 9/11 video

John Sferazo is an ironworker who rushed to Ground Zero as soon as he saw the towers burning. He worked long hours for the first few days, helping to cut up the massive iron beams. Even after he had to return to his regular construction job, he went to Ground Zero after he left his regular job each day in order to spend several hours helping to cut through the debris. He spent twenty-nine days working on the pile, not without lasting damage to his health:

> After breathing in all that toxic dust, I started getting repeated lung infections and pneumonia. Now I have reactive airway disease and what they call COPD, chronic obstructive pulmonary disease. I don't know if I can ever hold any kind of a real job now.
>
> I was in such good shape prior to 9/11. I could climb columns— that was part of my life when I was building skyscrapers. You have to have a high upper-body ratio to your mass weight to be able to pull yourself up a column and to do that continually, up repeated floors, and I had no problem doing that whatsoever. Today I don't even think about going up the stairs that are set on a job site to get to the upper elevations.

Part II, p. 113

Like so many others who were exposed to the Ground Zero toxins, John is now sensitive to a wide array of common chemical substances:

> Since 9/11, the smell of gasoline and diesel fuel bothers me so much that I don't get out and even fuel my own vehicles. I don't even want that stuff on my hands because of the odor. Being around the job sites and being around the smell of the diesel and gasoline, I was constantly getting problems with my throat. I would wind up going hoarse, and I would lose my voice. . . .
>
> Now I get headaches and burning in my lungs when I smell cigarette smoke, even though I used to work all the time in an

environment in which you would smell welders burning welding wire or burners cutting through iron. Since 9/11, the smell of smoke sometimes makes me gag or feel like throwing up.

I can't use many types of cologne or aftershave. I can't take that smell; it causes a burning feeling inside my nostrils. I notice now that some types of cologne have a very, very strong, pungent odor to them. Wherever I smell that kind of smell, I just have to get away from it.

Part II, p. 113

John Sferazo has become a major spokesperson for the people sickened by the 9/11 toxins, walking the halls of Congress to bring attention to this problem. He has appeared widely on New York and national television and was given an extensive time slot on "The Jim Lehrer News Hour" on the fifth anniversary of 9/11. John's health problems continue to be major. In the spring of 2008, he once again developed pneumonia, which has happened to him frequently since 9/11.

Kelly Colangelo lived in an apartment close to Ground Zero but was working in New Jersey when the terrorist attack on the Twin Towers occurred. She managed to enter her apartment briefly on September 12.

When I got into my apartment, it looked like it was snowing when I walked in. I had left my windows open, and the dust was about four inches thick on the window sills. Everything was covered in dust—sofa, rugs, toaster oven, coffee maker. . . . I quickly changed my clothes, put a few things in a suitcase, and left.

On the morning of September 14, I had a terrible headache. I was getting a sore throat, and later that day I started having this deep, throaty cough that sounded like I had been a chain smoker for fifteen years.

The following weekend I tried to get back to my apartment again. I ended up waiting most of the day on Johns Street with other residents of my building. We stood for hours breathing in that dust that was coming down like snow. They never did let us back into our building to get anything, so I checked into a hotel. That's when the fatigue hit me, just a constant fatigue. I couldn't walk up and down the subway stairs without having shortness of breath. I continued to have coughing fits and an awful headache.

. . . . . .

A few years after 9/11 I noticed that I was becoming very sensitive to certain smells like perfumes, colognes, cigarette smoke, and diesel fuel. When I walk down the sidewalk and somebody is smoking, I could just scream. I just can't stand the smell anymore. When someone is wearing too much cologne, I have to get away from them. I hold my breath now when I walk by buses because the diesel smell is too much for me to handle and gives me a headache.

Part II, pp. 266-69

Rachel Hughes was a young woman who volunteered to help unload trucks and pass out sandwiches to workers at Ground Zero. She would pay dearly for that act of compassion and patriotism, as she describes in her story that appears in Part II and in *The Toxic Clouds of 9/11*:

Within days of the 9/11 attacks, I had a fever and a constant headache; I was also vomiting and feeling dizzy. A bad cough made it hard for me to sleep. I was also having trouble breathing and had considerable chest pain and tightness. One of my worst problems was that large, unsightly sores started erupting on my scalp, face, neck, arms, and back. . . .

About a week after 9/11, I returned to work at my office, which was located about eight blocks north of the Trade Towers. . . . There was still thick dust all over our office, so we had to help clean our work spaces ourselves. I wore a surgical mask to work for several weeks because the air smelled horrible and was so thick with dust that it was hard to breathe, despite the assurances from the head of the EPA that the air was safe to breathe. . . . Even three months later the smoke in the area was still thick and made my eyes sting. Despite all the smoke and dust and fumes, I continued to work full-time in Lower Manhattan until I was laid off in December 2001 because of the negative effect 9/11 had on business.

My health problems related to the 9/11 toxic exposures have steadily worsened. I frequently have pneumonia or bronchitis. . . . Daily headaches are a problem, and I continue to have constant chest pain and pressure. My diagnoses include lung scarring.

Chemical sensitivity became a significant problem for me after my exposure to 9/11 toxins. Since that point, I have become sensitive to all types of chemical fumes that never gave me any problems before. I have had to stop wearing perfume and start using unscented body lotion and shampoo. The chemicals like ammonia or solvents that they use to clean the elevator or halls in my building make it difficult for me to breathe and sometimes give me a migraine. I actually try to hold my breath in the elevator because the cleaning products affect me so strongly.

I have always been a dedicated artist, but I can't paint right now because I'm too sensitive to the paint, even water-based paint. I'm too sensitive to markers to use them for illustration and drawing. The room in my apartment where I used to do art work after I could no longer afford to rent my art studio has turned into a medical billing station containing files of medical and insurance records.

Part II, pp. 139-41

Bonnie Giebfried was an emergency medical technician who was among the first ambulance crews responding to the terrorist attack. She was heavily exposed to the toxic dust when she barely escaped the huge mass of debris and dust that rolled through the area when each tower collapsed. Her health deteriorated so sharply that she had to give up her EMT job.

I had never had asthma before 9/11, but by the end of the day I had had three bad asthma attacks. That feeling of not being able to catch your breath, not being able to fill your lungs, is such a horrible, horrible feeling. It feels like someone's crushing your chest, sucking everything out of you. . . .

Before 9/11, I was in great health. I was playing on three soccer teams, three softball teams, a racquet ball league, a paddle ball league. I was fishing, hiking, climbing mountains. . . . I can't even climb up stairs now. I just can't catch my breath. I have chronic sinusitis, bronchitis, asthma. I just got over having pneumonia for the third time. Never had pneumonia before 9/11.

. . . . . .

Since 9/11, I've become very sensitive to various chemicals that never used to bother me, so I have to be really careful what I expose myself to. The other night I went out for Japanese food, which is one of my favorite things to do. I was having a good time with my life partner when this guy came in who was wearing a lot of cologne. My throat started closing up, and I began to get chest pains. I had to leave the restaurant, which was really disappointing. On other occasions, perfume exposure in a restaurant has caused me to become nauseated. . . . The multiple chemical sensitivity issues that have come from 9/11 have not been addressed.

I can't do normal, everyday things because of my chemical sensitivity. I really have to police myself to make sure that I'm not going to be exposed to gas fumes or the propane for the barbeque. Household cleaners, oh, my God, you just might as well pack me up at that point and send me to the hospital.

Part II, pp. 165-66

Alex Sanchez, his mother Iris, and friend Manuel are also among the many New Yorkers who developed multiple chemical sensitivity after they were exposed to the WTC toxins. Alex Sanchez said when we filmed him, "We have problems with getting into places where there's lots of chemicals or heavy perfume." In particular, he said that he has trouble with the perfume exposures he encounters on a subway, which means that he has to use his scarce resources to take a cab to medical appointments.

When one realizes that exposure to something like the burning oil wells in Kuwait or the WTC fires will almost certainly induce chemical sensitivity in a significant percentage of those exposed, it is frustrating to simply watch it happen when knowledge about MCS could reduce the downward spiral in these people's health. I realized right away on 9/11 that not only were many residents of the Ground Zero area going to develop chemical sensitivity, but many would also decide to move to an apartment farther away from Ground Zero. That was a decision that could bring its own problems because chemically sensitive people almost always react to new paint and new carpet, elements that one often encounters in a new rental but may be avoidable if one is aware of the potential problem.

At one meeting about 9/11 health problems that I attended on Long Island, a woman whose husband is now chronically ill asked me if her burning of scented candles throughout the house could be increasing her husband's breathing problems. It's clear that sick people and their families need to be given information about how to reduce exposure to substances that may cause asthma attacks or give them headaches.

An interesting case in point is that of a woman whose story appears in Part II under her initials, H. D. When we filmed her in early 2006 for *The Toxic Clouds of 9/11*, I asked her if she had developed any chemical sensitivity along with her other post-9/11 health problems. She replied that she had not, but when I spoke to her a year later, she said that once I had alerted her to the issue, she began to notice that her asthma attacks were often triggered by chemical exposures.

Dr. Stephen Levin spoke in my 9/11 documentary about the unusual reactions that WTC patients were reporting to him:

> Another striking thing is that many of our patients are much more reactive to strong odors than they were before. . . . I have patients who cannot walk into a department store cosmetic area without experiencing shortness of breath and chest tightness in ways they never did before. I have patients who cannot get on an elevator where someone is wearing strong perfume or cologne without experiencing fairly intense respiratory reactions. We don't always understand why this is so, but it is extremely commonly reported among our World Trade Center responders and many of our patients say that they are simply unable to wear fragrances themselves or be around others–family members, friends–who wear such fragrances because they simply can't tolerate them.

There are obviously major health problems that large numbers of New Yorkers are facing as the result of the terrible toxic exposures near Ground Zero. Knowledge of chemical sensitivity isn't going to prevent someone from developing leukemia or lung cancer or mesothelioma, but avoidance of chemical exposures can for many of these sick people reduce the headaches, joint pains, fatigue, asthma, and other symptoms that are currently making their lives difficult.

Chapter 8

Katrina's Toxic Aftermath

Hurricane Katrina's torrential wind and rain left a swath of widespread destruction in an area covered by petroleum refineries, chemical processing plants, and pesticide factories. The September 26, 2005, issue of *Business Week* referred to the challenge of dealing with the tons and tons of "lethal goop" left behind by Katrina as the "mother of all toxic cleanups." As the result of the hurricane's destruction, many toxic chemicals were released into the ground, air, and water, and the long-term health consequences are an urgent issue that few government agencies are addressing.

An article appearing in the British newspaper *The Independent* on September 11, 2005, stated:

> Other US sources spelt out the extent of the danger from one of America's most polluted industrial areas, known locally as "Cancer Alley." The 66 chemical plants, refineries and petroleum storage depots churn out 600m lb of toxic waste each year. Other dangerous substances are in site storage tanks or at the port of New Orleans. No one knows how much pollution has escaped through damaged plants and leaking pipes into the "toxic gumbo" now drowning the city.

Hugh Kaufman, who helped found the EPA and has worked for decades in the area of toxic waste and Superfund sites, is particularly concerned about the Katrina situation, as he stated on the "Jim Lehrer Newshour" on September 19, 2005:

> You have got cancer-causing chemicals from the petrochemical industry that are in the muck and in the water. I think the decision to bring people back into the city without doing an assessment of the–how much toxicity is there, is just reckless and irresponsible.

In one notable example, over a million gallons of fuel escaped from the Murphy Oil Refinery, contaminating a nearby residential area in St. Bernard Parish, which borders New Orleans.[1] In its report "Katrina's Wake," which describes the release of toxic substances resulting from the hurricane's fury, the Natural Resources Defense Council has documented the many oil spills that occurred in the area:

> According to the U.S. Coast Guard and the EPA, some 575 Katrina-related spills of petroleum or hazardous chemicals were reported in the aftermath of the storm. Ten major to medium oil spills have fouled the Mississippi River from Chalmette to Venice and west to Port Fourchon, releasing a total of nearly 8 million gallons of oil, and the Coast Guard estimates that the region endured approximately 124 minor spills of less than 10,000 gallons each . . . The flood-affected area has some 2,200 underground fuel tanks, an unknown percentage of which ruptured in the storm. [2]

The nearly eight million gallons of oil released in Louisiana by Katrina's destructive force constitute the next largest oil spill in U.S. history after the *Exxon Valdez* disaster, which according to Exxon released just under eleven million gallons. Given the huge media attention to potential environmental consequences following the *Exxon Valdez* spill, it seems surprising that more attention has not been paid to the health problems that so much spilled oil could be causing to residents of Louisiana.

One newspaper, the *Dallas Morning News,* did address this issue in a November 6, 2005, article titled "Massive Effort Planned to Deal with Toxins Deposited in Soil by Flood." Environmental reporter Randy Lee Loftis described the results of chemical tests the EPA had conducted through October 1 in Orleans Parish, whose boundaries coincide with the city of New Orleans. One particularly alarming result, according to

---

[1] Natural Resources Defense Council report, "Katrina's Wake," August 2007, p. 17, www.nrdc.org/health/effects/wake/contents.asp.

[2] "Katrina's Wake," p. 16.

Loftis, was that "About 150 residential test sites had as much diesel as the soil around a leaking underground tank."

The Natural Resources Defense Council's "Katrina's Wake" report states that some locations in the Chalmette and St. Roch neighborhoods near New Orleans "had diesel fuel contamination more than 200 times the Louisiana soil-cleanup level."[3] In fact, over ninety percent of the samples that the EPA conducted in Uptown/Carrolton, Central City/Garden, Mid-City, Gentilly, Bywater, New Orleans East, and Arabi in St. Bernard Parish tested in excess of the standards in place to trigger soil-cleanup by the state. According to the NRDC, there were "eight hot spots where levels of diesel-range organics are more than 100 times higher than the LDEQ [Louisiana Department of Environmental Quality] soil cleanup and investigation standard for residential neighborhoods."[4]

In a related problem, some 350,000 cars or other vehicles were ruined in the floods, potentially releasing millions of gallons of gasoline or oil into the floodwaters and ultimately the sediment that was left coating residential yards and playgrounds. The leader of the NRDC team, Gina Solomon, M.D., warned that "Residents face a health risk because they can easily inhale contaminated sediment or get it on their skin when they are trying to clean it up."[5]

Petroleum products were not the only major source of pollution. Significant amounts of pesticides ended up in the floodwaters. Some came from pesticide supplies that were sitting in people's garages when the hurricane swept through, destroying many buildings in residential areas. One particularly bad pesticide exposure occurred near the Gert Town neighborhood of Mid-City in New Orleans. Gert Town was unfortunately close to an abandoned plant where pesticides were formerly produced. To compound the problem, pesticides had often been mixed on the grounds around the plant, so the soil was contaminated.

---

[3] "Katrina's Wake," p. 13.

[4] NRDC press release, February 23, 2006, "NRDC Analyzes EPA Sediment Data," www.nrdc.org/health/effects/katrinadata/contents.asp.

[5] Ibid.

Tests of soil samples conducted by the Natural Resources Defense Council and Dr. Wilma Subra, a Louisiana chemist who specializes in environmental issues, found dangerous levels of pesticides near this facility. One sample taken close to some homes bordering the plant contained DDT at a level twice that which should trigger a cleanup according to the EPA and dieldrin at a level almost seven times that which would trigger a cleanup. According to the NRDC, DDT and dieldrin "are suspected human carcinogens, have been linked to neurological problems and hormonal system disruption, have been banned in the United States for more than 25 years, and are now banned worldwide by international treaty."[6]

The NRDC also raised the alarm about the dangerous levels of mold found throughout Katrina's path of destruction. According to Dr. Solomon, "The outdoor mold spore concentrations could easily trigger serious allergic or asthmatic reactions in sensitive people. The indoor air quality was even worse, rendering the homes we tested dangerously uninhabitable by any definition."[7] In addition to the problem of allergic reactions to mold that are mediated by IgE antibodies, many people also react to the toxic chemicals called mycotoxins that molds give off.

Because of the widespread contamination from toxic chemicals and heavy metals as well as mold, the NRDC and other environmental groups were urging returning residents to wear special full-body protective suits and use respirators. Joel Shufro, who is the Executive Director of the New York Committee for Occupational Safety and Health, raised such concerns:

There are very serious chemical and respiratory hazards throughout the areas affected by Hurricanes Katrina and Rita. Exposure to those hazards without proper protection can cause serious life-long health problems. . . . To help people in need is noble,

---

[6] Ibid.

[7] Ibid.

but I would urge young people to make certain that they will not
be seriously compromising their health while doing so.[8]

Unfortunately, such cautionary messages apparently did not reach most
of the volunteer groups. Once again, as in the aftermath of 9/11, gener-
ous and idealistic people who wanted to help others in a time of crisis
risked their own health because government agencies such as the EPA
failed to raise the alarm about the toxic substances present in the floodwaters, sediment, and mold that had coated people's yards and their
homes.

Alex Rubin was an idealistic junior high student from Newton,
Massachusetts, who went down to Louisiana with his mother and
several other volunteers to help clean the hurricane-damaged houses
during his spring vacation. When he entered the house they were
assigned to work on, he was shocked by what he saw:

> The carpet was still sopping wet over four months after Hurricane
> Rita. Everything in sight was covered with green, red, black and
> white mold. . . . The first thing I saw in the dim light was the
> couch. It had mold growing all over it, top to bottom. Before we
> could clean the walls, we had to take everything out of the house.
> . . . Everything I touched was infested with mold and smelled
> terrible. As we carried moldy things out to the street, mold got in
> our hair and in our clothes.[9]

The inevitable result of the toxic exposures faced by volunteers and
residents of the Gulf States is that a sizable percentage of those exposed
will have developed multiple chemical sensitivity. Anyone who was
aware of MCS shuddered when they heard that people who lost their
homes in the hurricane were going to be housed in trailers provided by
FEMA because people who have developed chemical sensitivity almost
always find it hard to tolerate living in trailers, which have substantial

---

[8] "Student Volunteers at Risk in Gulf Coast: What Students and Other Young
Volunteers Can Do to Help Without Risking Their Health," by Ellie Goldberg,
M.Ed., www.healthy-kids.info.

[9] www.wickedlocal.com/newton/archive/x902753599.

levels of formaldehyde because of the insulation, paneling, subflooring, and particleboard cabinets and furniture, all contained in a small, confined space.

On its Indoor Air Quality website, the EPA discusses formaldehyde and the health effects it can cause:

> Formaldehyde, a colorless, pungent-smelling gas, can cause watery eyes, burning sensations in the eyes and throat, nausea, and difficulty in breathing in some humans exposed at elevated levels (above 0.1 parts per million). High concentrations may trigger attacks in people with asthma. There is evidence that some people can develop a sensitivity to formaldehyde. It has also been shown to cause cancer in animals and may cause cancer in humans. Health effects include eye, nose, and throat irritation; wheezing and coughing; fatigue; skin rash; severe allergic reactions. May cause cancer.[10]

Given the known dangers of exposure to formaldehyde, it was particularly egregious that FEMA housed the Katrina refugees in travel trailers, which are not meant for long-term occupancy and contain even higher levels of formaldehyde than mobile homes. As a result, large numbers of FEMA trailer residents are now sick, and the elderly and children have been especially hard hit.

Lindsay Huckabee testified on July 19, 2007, to the House Government Reform and Oversight Committee chaired by Henry A. Waxman about her family's experience in a FEMA trailer:

> As we were moving into the trailer, we noticed that it had a very strong odor. We figured that is what a "new" trailer smelled like. Our whole family began to have sinus problems, our eyes would burn and water, and our throats were constantly sore. We seemed to catch every cold and virus going around, but we couldn't get rid of the illnesses. Three of our children began having severe nosebleeds, sometimes three or four times a week. I began having migraine headaches and pre-term labor. . . .

---

[10] www.epa.gov/iaq/formalde.html.

Over the next 18 months, Lelah [four at the time] had more ear infections than I can count, nosebleeds several times a month, sometimes as many as a three a week. She had pneumonia several times. For most of the cases, she was treated at home with steroids and breathing treatments, but she had to be hospitalized twice because the pneumonia was so severe.

After months and months of office visits and phone calls, I was frustrated and upset. I came home one afternoon to find my daughter covering her nose; her hands, arms and shirt were covered in blood. The surprising part is that I did not feel the need to rush to her and find out what was wrong. I did not think for a second that it was anything more than a bloody nose. Two years ago, I would have panicked trying to get to her. Later that night, I cried for hours. How had we gotten to the point where I was not surprised to see my child covered in blood?

Part II, pp. 228-30

The experience of the Huckabee family seems hardly surprising, given the information about the dangers of formaldehyde exposure that appears on the website of the Agency for Toxic Substances and Disease Registry (ATSDR), a subagency of the U.S. Department of Health and Human Services:

Formaldehyde is an eye, skin, and respiratory tract irritant. Inhalation of vapors can produce narrowing of the bronchi and an accumulation of fluid in the lungs. Children may be more susceptible than adults to the respiratory effects of formaldehyde. Formaldehyde solution (formalin) causes corrosive injury to the gastrointestinal tract, especially the pharynx, epiglottis, esophagus, and stomach. . . . Even fairly low concentrations of formaldehyde can produce rapid onset of nose and throat irritation, causing cough, chest pain, shortness of breath, and wheezing. Higher exposures can cause significant inflammation of the lower respiratory tract, resulting in swelling of the throat, inflammation of the windpipe and bronchi, narrowing of the bronchi, inflammation of the lungs, and accumulation of fluid in the lungs. . . . Children may be more vulnerable to corrosive agents than adults because of the relatively smaller diameter of their airways.

Children may be more vulnerable because of relatively increased minute ventilation per kg.[11]

The pertinence of the ATSDR warnings about the dangers of exposure to formaldehyde is clear from Lindsay Huckabee's testimony to the House Science and Technology Committee on April 1, 2008, when she again described the health problems that each of her five children had had after moving into their FEMA trailer. She was particularly concerned about the trailer's effect on her two-year-old son, who was born prematurely after they moved into their trailer. She had carried all four of her other children to term or past term.

> Michael has had sinus infections off and on since he was six days old; he has also had asthmatic bronchitis, pneumonia, laryngitis, only a few nosebleeds and undergone cardiac testing because he occasionally turns blue for an unknown reason. Michael is currently on two daily allergy medications, a nasal steroid, and antibiotics for the sixth straight week. Michael has been hospitalized three times.
>
> Part II, pp. 233

The enormity of the family health problems that Lindsay has been dealing with is illustrated by her testimony that her son Steven "has been pretty fortunate health wise." Perhaps this was because he had only been hospitalized once. She did tell the committee members that since living in the trailer, "He has had asthmatic bronchitis, pneumonia, sinus infections and nosebleeds."

There have been other reports of babies who lived in FEMA trailers turning blue. Wanda Phillips, whose story appears in Part II, describes the experience of a daughter who was living with her in a FEMA trailer several days a week while she was pregnant.

> I worry especially about my youngest granddaughter because my daughter had such difficulty carrying her. By the time she was three-months-old, my granddaughter had had a couple of spells where she quit breathing and her legs from the knees down turned blue. In my research, I have found that there are documented

---

[11] "Medical Management Guidelines for Formaldehyde," ATSDR website, www.atsdr.cdc.gov/MHMI/mmg111.html.

cases of birth defects caused by exposure to formaldehyde in the first trimester of pregnancy. My daughter lived with me for three or four days every week during her pregnancy and still continues to stay with me. She and my granddaughters also stayed with me in our FEMA trailer. My daughter had recurrent labor for weeks before her daughter was born. She took medications for the problem and was admitted to the hospital on more than one occasion to stop her from giving birth too early. Even then she delivered her baby early.

Part II, p. 133

The House Committee on Oversight and Government Reform has heard not only from individuals like Lindsay Huckabee but also from the CEO's of various companies that supplied the travel trailers, as well as from some employees of one company. In its majority staff report, the Oversight Committee discussed testing that was carried out by the Gulf Stream company, which had signed a contract with FEMA to provide over 50,000 travel trailers:

Gulf Stream discovered high levels of formaldehyde concentrations in trailers they had manufactured and also in trailers made by other manufacturers. Every occupied trailer tested had levels above 100 ppb [0.1 ppm], the level at which CDC, the Environmental Protection Agency (EPA), the World Health Organization, the Consumer Product Safety Commission, and the National Institute of Occupational Safety and Health say acute adverse health effects can be experienced. Four of the 11 occupied trailers had levels above 500 ppb, the level at which federal occupational safety regulations require medical monitoring for worker exposure. . . . [O]ver 20 unoccupied trailers had formaldehyde levels above 900 ppb, a level at which EPA says it is dangerous to be exposed for more than eight hours in a lifetime, with several trailers having levels above 2,000 ppb.[12]

----

[12] House Committee on Oversight and Government Reform, Majority Staff Analysis, "Trailer Manufacturers and Elevated Formaldehyde Levels," July 9, 2008, www.oversight.house.gov/documents/20080709103125.pdf, p. 2.

The Waxman committee grilled FEMA executives about what has become known as the "toxic trailer" issue. One committee report relates the following shocking information:

> FEMA testing of a trailer occupied by a pregnant mother and her infant in April 2006–apparently the only occupied FEMA trailer ever tested by FEMA–showed formaldehyde levels that were 75 times higher than the maximum workplace exposure level recommended by the National Institute for Occupational Safety and Health.
>
> Despite the evidence of a formaldehyde problem in FEMA trailers, FEMA officials in headquarters, acting on the advice of FEMA lawyers, refused to test occupied FEMA trailers. One FEMA attorney explained: "Do not initiate any testing until we give the OK. . . . Once you get results and should they indicate some problem, the clock is running on our duty to respond to them." [13]

The House Oversight Committee also interviewed two former Gulf Stream employees. Linda Esparza said they had worked "15-hour days with a frantic production schedule . . . There would be supervisors and plant managers walking down the line with bullhorns screaming at us, go faster, you're not doing your job, you don't deserve your pay-check."[14] Gulf Stream's co-presidents got very good paychecks out of their frenzied FEMA trailer production; the salary for each doubled during that period.[15]

Terry Slone, who was in charge of flooring installation in the Gulf Stream trailers, told the Oversight Committee: "you were expected to

---

[13] House Committee on Oversight and Governmental Reform, Hurricane Katrina Response, Supplemental Memo and Exhibits, "Committee Probes FEMA's Response to Reports of Toxic Trailers," July 19, 2007.

[14] House Committee on Oversight and Government Reform, Majority Staff Analysis, "Trailer Manufacturers and Elevated Formaldehyde Levels," July 9, 2008, www.oversight.house.gov/documents/20080709103125.pdf, p. 10.

[15] Ibid., p. 19.

work as hard and as fast as you could." The adverse health effects that he experienced included nosebleeds, shortness of breath, dizziness, and bleeding from his ears. Linda Esparza said that it felt as if she had a "sinus infection that lasted the whole time I was there."[16]

Terry told the House Oversight Committee that he realized that the foul odor in the plant was being emitted by the manufactured wood products they were using in the travel trailers because when he would lift a piece of wood material off a pile, the odor "was just overwhelming." Linda Esparza noted that "workers could not stay in one of the recently completed travel trailers for 'maybe 5 or 10 minutes before your eyes were watering and your nose was burning.'"[17] Her son, Tommy Yager, helped lay floorboards in the trailers. Tommy and Linda appeared in a July 8, 2008, segment on "CBS Evening News" that was devoted to the toxic trailer problem. A former EMT, Tommy reported, "We had guys that would have such bad flu symptoms they'd drop right on the floor. . . . just keel over." According to Linda, Gulf Stream knew that there was a formaldehyde problem with the trailers:

> FEMA would show up around 9 or 10 in the morning to do their inspections. About a couple hours before they came out to do their inspection, we were instructed to open the doors and windows so the odor wouldn't be as strong when the inspectors got there.[18]

Because there was such a rush to push as many trailers as possible off the assembly line, many companies used plywood and particleboard from China and other Asian countries that contained very high levels of formaldehyde. In an October 8, 2008, article titled "U.S. Rules Allow the Sale of Products Others Ban," the *Los Angeles Times* stated:

> Though China sends low-formaldehyde timber to Japan and Europe, Americans are getting wood that emits substantially higher levels of the chemical. One birch plank from China,

---

[16] Ibid., pp. 10-11.

[17] Ibid., p. 11

[18] "RV Workers React to Congressional Hearings on Toxic Trailers," WSBT2 TV, South Bend, Indiana, July 9, 2008,

bought at a Home Depot store in Portland, gave off 100 times more formaldehyde than legal in Japan and 30 times more than allowed in Europe and China.

Yet another alarming statement about formaldehyde comes from an article that appeared in the *Washington Post* on July 3, 2008:

> The CDC recommended this year that all FEMA trailer residents be moved to safer housing. The agency found that 42 percent of trailers tested in December and January had levels of formaldehyde higher than those for which it recommends a 15-minute exposure limit for workers.

What makes the FEMA trailer situation especially tragic is that it is not unlikely that large numbers of the trailer residents who have become sick will now react to other chemicals that they encounter in their everyday life, such as paint, perfume, auto exhaust, cigarette smoke, diesel fumes, and air fresheners. For those who have developed multiple chemical sensitivity, they will unfortunately find that this condition will have a significant impact upon their lives. It is particularly sad to think of the little children who have been sensitized to the chemicals they will encounter throughout the rest of their lives. Lynn Henderson describes the effect living in a FEMA trailer has had on two little girls she is raising because their mother was killed in an auto accident:

> The three-year-old and the seventeen-month-old baby are now very sensitive to all sorts of scented products. I started noticing that when I would put on body lotion after my shower and then walk by the baby, she would sneeze over and over again until she was out of breath. Then in a minute she would start sneezing again. I can't wear perfume any more because it bothers the little girls so much, and they also react to hair spray and cleaning products I use.
>
> Part II, p. 189

The chemical sensitivity induced in these little girls will almost certainly cause very troublesome problems as they enter the school system and eventually the workforce. This is a heavy responsibility for the federal government, which failed in an abysmal way these children and other trailer residents.

FEMA not only carries a substantial moral burden at this point; the agency is also facing lawsuits on behalf of 800 named plaintiffs who lived in the "toxic" trailers. Their lawyers are arguing that many of the trailers the agency provided to Gulf Coast residents after Hurricanes Katrina and Rita contained unsafe levels of formaldehyde. On October 3, 2008, the Associated Press published an article titled "Judge: FEMA not immune from toxic trailer suits" that stated:

> U.S. District Judge Kurt Engelhardt cited evidence that the Federal Emergency Management Agency delayed investigating complaints about formaldehyde levels in its trailers because it might be held legally responsible.

FEMA's reprehensible policy of not acting quickly once it learned about the high formaldehyde levels in the trailers it was providing to people has exposed the federal government and taxpayers to enormous potential costs because of the damage that has occurred to the health of so many Gulf Coast residents who never dreamed that the government would offer them housing that would destroy their health. And the 800 named plaintiffs in the current lawsuits are only the tip of the iceberg. FEMA provided over 143,000 trailers to Gulf Coast residents, with an average of three residents per trailer, according a statement made by the administrator of FEMA, R. David Paulison, in a February 14, 2008, press conference. That means that the health of over 400,000 people has been potentially been put at risk.

The parallels to the handling of the World Trade Center disaster cleanup by city, state, and federal governments are painfully apparent. The WTC lawsuit involving over 10,000 workers has government officials concerned about the huge financial outlay that may result from this lawsuit. As with FEMA, the problem is that government officials paid insufficient attention to potentially toxic situations. At some point, America's leaders must realize that their refusal to take toxic exposures seriously is in the long run a costly mistake that engenders not only potentially large legal settlements but also creates a group of citizens whose health is so impaired that they will need public assistance to get through life.

Part II

John Sferazo

9/11 Ironworker

I spent much of my earlier years in the Big Woods of northwestern Maine and the Adirondack Mountains of New York. It was easy to love the outdoors because this was where I found solace and serenity. Hunting, fishing, trapping, hiking, and camping came easy to me and became my truest passion. I was raised to respect all our Great Spirit created and to only take what you need from Mother Earth and always give back to her. She is there to nurture you if you understand a simpler life style. I was very fortunate to have a Native American influence in my upbringing, and I give thanks for this. As time passed and I grew older, however, I left this simple life style in Maine and moved to New York, where I started a new life as a union ironworker. I helped build New York City skyscrapers; this became my new life.

Then the terrorist attacks happened, changing my life forever. My career as an ironworker was soon to be over because my physical condition changed so dramatically, in such a short time. I had formerly been healthy except for a back injury and was proud of not missing any time from work except in an emergency. That all changed with 9/11. By early 2002, I was missing more and more days at work. By the time I left my job on August 1, 2004, my new medical ailments had forced me to miss over a hundred days of work.

On the morning of 9/11, I was working for a construction outfit on a rehabilitation project on the Marine Park Bridge, which connects Long Island to Rockaway. I was working directly over the water, and of course sound carries very well when there are no obstructions blocking it. To this day, I can still hear the rumbling of the first tower as it collapsed. Being ironworkers in the construction field, where every day you face danger, my fellow workers and I knew we had to go to the World Trade Center site and do whatever we could to help. Ironworkers not only build these structures, we also take them down. This job had our name on it and was what we were used to doing. As everyone else was running from this tragedy, we rushed in to help our fellow man. I will always remember the sight of all of us running to answer a beckoning call from Lady Liberty herself in the harbor nearby. It made me proud to be an American—courage runs in our blood.

We mobilized our equipment, trying to be sure to take all we would need for what might lie ahead as we waited for permission to enter this disaster zone. Early on the morning of September 12, we finally received word to enter Manhattan through the Battery Tunnel. It had taken all night for the city's structural engineers to verify the tunnel's capacity to support our passage with all the heavy equipment we were bringing with us. A police escort was waiting for us to arrive at the entrance to the tunnel, where we joined with various police and fire department units that were also heading to Ground Zero with all their equipment.

Some things in life never leave you, and most of what I witnessed in those days after the terrorist attack will forever remain imbedded in my memory. Those memories are so intense that I can still smell that smell of death and can still hear the sound of the sirens ringing in my ears. I can see the fighter jets making a flyover, the helicopters hovering overhead, and the unbelievable destruction all around us. After we entered West Street, we started coming to grips with the reality of everything we were seeing. Some of us got out of our vehicles and kneeled on the sidewalk next to the trucks to say a fast prayer and make the sign of the cross.

Backing our tractor-trailer trucks up to the first piece of blocking debris in this huge quagmire of wreckage, we started using hydraulically operated booms to clear the streets leading to Ground Zero. We moved wrecked vehicles of all types and sizes, chunks of concrete and iron locked together, and pieces of rebar and wire that were tangled together. As I was working, I suddenly saw right in front of me the very piece of reality that had caused this massive heap of debris—a fragment of an airplane. I wept in silence as I retrieved it and walked up to a policeman to ask him what to do with it. I knew there would be time to think about this at some later point, but right now I knew there could be some people who were still alive trapped in this huge pile of rubble. The very last thing on your mind at a time like this is your own safety because all around you is reality the likes of which you have never experienced before.

We cleared the streets up to a flooded location that was very close to where the South Tower had been. There was a small pool there because right after the attack the New York Fire Department had been instructed to spray water on the cooling tank below the South Tower to keep it from overheating and possibly exploding. At first, we had no idea that we were looking at a large pool of water because the surface was covered with what looked like oatmeal. This was the powdery remnants of various construction materials. To this day, we have no idea what toxic chemicals we may have absorbed through our skin when we waded through pools of water like this.

All around us a thick cloud of fine fibers and particles was floating in the air. It was so thick that you could almost cut it with a knife. When there were slight gusts of wind, an even thicker cloud of dust would float by and engulf you, causing you to tear-up and choke uncontrollably. We kept coughing out chunks of debris and dust that we couldn't avoid breathing in or swallowing.

After clearing West Street as far as that new pond on that first day we were there, we had to wait for our oxygen tanks to be delivered so that we could start cutting up the iron beams with our acetylene torches. In the meantime, a bucket brigade started moving debris off the pile. I helped do this for a while until I saw a police officer with a search-and-rescue dog. Since I had been trained and certified in wild land search-and-rescue by the NYC Department of Environmental Conservation, I asked the policeman if I could accompany him and his dog. Having been on the gymnastic team and the track team in high school, I was very agile and could follow the dog into the deep holes that he entered. Wherever there was a hollow in this immense pile, that was where this dog would nose around.

Sometimes the dog and I went down several floors below street level, almost like we were exploring some dark cave. I remember that one time I had to lie down with my back against the web of a column that was now lying flat in this pile and use the column flange overhead to guide me as I followed the dog. As I worked myself further and further down into this debris, with only a small flashlight to guide me, I had to pull myself over pieces of electrical conduit and pipes. Every now and then I would become entangled in something. I kept thinking that the wreckage above me might collapse on top of me at any moment. At least during the daytime, I could see a little light at the end of the "tunnels" I had climbed into, but at night I didn't even have that to guide me in retracing my steps and had to rely solely on my flashlight.

I worked with the policeman and his dog for only six or seven hours, but it seemed like a lifetime. When the dog found what he was after, he lay down next to it and looked at me or barked. The worse thing this dog found was what was left of a man's head, and I could only tell that when I put the light on it. I had to carry it out of the pile to hand it over to a group collecting human remains, and I still have nightmares about carrying that piece of a man's head. I doubt if those dreams will ever leave me, and thinking about that horrible experience brings tears to my eyes to this day. The things we witnessed and the experiences we endured have left us with mental scarring. I had problems defusing what I saw at Ground Zero, so I went to a trauma counselor for help. I was taught how to focus on this horrible event and the nightmares that plague me and make them turn out better and more acceptable in my imagination, but it took me a long time to learn how to do that. Like so many other First Responders, in addition to major respiratory problems, I suffer from PTSD (post-traumatic stress disorder). I pray that this PTSD will someday go away, but I don't know if it will.

In several spots we were working, the dog and I were inhaling a green smoke. Later, I heard that the green smoke came predominately from burning computer screens. With all the toxins and chemicals on that burning pile, we wonder what we have inside us at this point.

After we had worked at Ground Zero for several days, we were sent back to our job on the Marine Park Bridge. But me and several other guys kept going back to the Trade Center site at night. And of course, the cops and the firemen loved to have us ironworkers there, so they didn't stop us from going into the site. We would work next to guys who were getting paid because this was their job. We weren't getting paid; we were there as volunteers, utilizing our capacity as ironworkers to cut up the enormous iron beams and columns, all the massive structures that were still there.

I knew something was wrong with my health even while I was still working at the World Trade Center. I had what most doctors called a WTC cough. Sometimes I would cough up sputum that was grey and blackish. Sometimes there was even blood mixed in, depending upon how hard I was coughing or what I had been exposed to. I had no respiratory problems prior to 9/11; I could even run a mile in five minutes and thirty seconds when I was on my high school track team. Then, after breathing in all that toxic dust, I started getting repeated lung infections and pneumonia. Now I have reactive airway disease and what they call COPD, chronic obstructive pulmonary disease. My other health issues include gastroesophageal reflux, chronic sinusitis, chronic breathing problems, and an extreme sleep apnea. I was recently told that my labored breathing is caused not just by lung damage from all the toxins I was exposed to but also by the stomach acid that comes up in my throat and then gets inside my lungs. Given all these health problems, I don't know if I can ever hold any kind of a real job now.

I was in such good shape prior to 9/11. I could climb columns—that was part of my life when I was building skyscrapers. You have to have a high upper-body ratio to your mass weight to be able to pull yourself up a column and to do that continually, up repeated floors, and I had no problem doing that. Today I don't even think about going up the stairs that are set on a job site to get to the upper elevations.

Since 9/11, the smell of gasoline and diesel fuel bothers me so much that I don't fuel my own vehicles. I don't even want that stuff on my hands because of the odor. Being around the job sites and being around the smell of the diesel and gasoline, I was constantly getting problems with my throat. I would wind up going hoarse, and I would lose my voice. I would go from a sore throat to a chest infection and then sometimes I would get pneumonia, and this had never ever happened to me before in my life.

Now I get headaches and burning in my lungs when I smell cigarette smoke, even though I used to work all the time in an environment in which you would smell welders burning welding wire or burners cutting through iron. Since 9/11, the smell of smoke sometimes makes me gag or feel like throwing up. I can't use cologne or aftershave. I can't take that smell; it causes a burning feeling inside my nostrils. I notice now that some types of cologne have a very, very strong, pungent odor to them. Wherever I smell that kind of smell, I just have to get away from it.

Before 9/11, I had an excellent job as a construction ironworker. It was challenging and kept my life interesting. You make an awful lot of friends as an ironworker, working outside with so many different trades. I made very decent money before I had to stop working in August of 2004. Now what I used to make in a day, I have to live on for a week.

Currently, I'm only getting workers' compensation at $400 a week, which doesn't go very far. If my wife wasn't helping to support me, I honestly don't know what position I'd be in.

Before the World Trade Center attack, I worked every single day and hour I could. I did all the overtime I could because I was paying child support for three children from my first marriage. But then after 9/11, I kept getting sick and would be out of work for several days at a time, so I wasn't able to earn what I used to. Eventually I had to give up working altogether.

There are thousands of people like me who became sick because of their 9/11 exposures, and they are falling through the cracks. They're not being given what's justly due them as far as workers' compensation, Social Security, and other benefits are concerned. As I've said in Washington, D.C., on several occasions, I feel like government officials are telling me that I'm expendable. Once I'm a liability, I'm no longer needed. They said they would never forget 9/11, but they have forgotten so many people like me who have become sick after 9/11. When the insurance companies do not want to pay their obligations and your government tries to sweep you under the rug, then it is only the strong and determined who continue to fight. I used to believe in my government, but now I am sorry to say that trust is gone.

We've become different people since 9/11. A lot of us, we explain it sometimes by saying that if you were dead it would have been a final saving grace in some respects but being left alive and symptomatic from what you experienced leaves you a hollow shell of an individual and you feel that way because it's not the same you.

Greta

Exxon Valdez Cleanup Worker

My parents were commercial fishermen in Cook Inlet, where they had their own boat. My sister and I usually spent summers fishing with them to earn money for college. The summer after the oil spill, when I was nineteen, Cook Inlet was polluted by the oil, so we weren't able to fish. My mom and my sister and I all got hired by VECO to help clean the beaches in July and August because they were looking for women to help fill their quota of minorities. A week or two later my dad joined us on the cleanup.

Before we left Valdez for the six- to eight-hour ferry ride to the barge where we were supposed to sleep at night, the people in charge held a safety meeting for us. They said we should make sure the oil didn't get on our skin. That turned out to be a joke because when we started working, we discovered it was impossible to keep the oil off our skin. To make the situation worse, there wasn't anywhere on the beaches where you could wash the oil off your hands before you ate.

They gave us boots, a helmet, rain gear, and plastic gloves, but we got a lot of oil on our faces. They gave us a can of foam stuff to put on our face and exposed skin, and my mom and sister and I used it. Others didn't. It probably came off when we sweat anyway.

When we reached the beach on the first day after riding for an hour from our berthing vessel, they assigned us to clean the rocks with pompoms, which were balls made of half-inch strips of plastic. We would sit down on the rocks while we were working because it was hard to bend down for hour after hour. There were fumes coming off the oily rocks, and between the rocks there were puddles of oil containing decaying seaweed that smelled really bad. I remember a couple of spots that smelled so terrible that we could only work there for a few minutes at a time. People were getting lightheaded and dizzy and nauseous from the oil fumes; sometimes we felt like we might pass out. They had to take one person off the beach because she was starting to hallucinate.

When our pom-poms got full of oil, we would put them into black plastic garbage bags. There must have been tons and tons of those garbage bags full of oily pom-poms. We always wondered how they were going to dispose of all those bags because every day we filled dozens of them.

We were always sitting in oil, and the odor would give us headaches. When we leaned down to work, oil would often splatter on our faces and sometimes our wrists would get exposed. We couldn't pull off our gloves to eat without ending up with oil on our hands and on our food. After you pulled off one glove, you had to pull the other glove off with your bare hand, so of course you ended up with oil all over that hand.

During the first couple of weeks, we were getting really dehydrated because the only way we could get a drink out of our bag was to take off our gloves, which was a messy operation. After a while, we started bringing water jugs and cups and some first-aid stuff. We finally got rebellious, so the supervisors let us set up a "safety station," where we kept a cooler with water in it and cups and snacks and first-aid supplies. My mom and sister worked that station, and it was great to be able to have a drink without having to take off your oily gloves. And when my glasses got oily, they would clean them for me.

At first there weren't even any bathroom facilities on the beaches. We just had to go out in the woods and take off our gear, which wasn't easy when it was covered with oil, so once again it was hard to keep the oil off our skin. Eventually they set up tents that contained something like port-a-potties.

On one of the beaches we were assigned to, we had to cross slippery rocks to reach the beach. That was really scary. One man fell and broke his leg, and an ambulance boat had to come for him. Most of us ended up crawling over the rocks.

I stopped working two weeks before my classes were supposed to start at the University of Anchorage. A year or so after the spill I started having horrible migraines; I had never had migraines before. After the cleanup, I also developed asthma. During the first year or so after the oil spill, I would get aching in the bones in my legs, which I had never had before, and my joints are painful now. I started noticing other changes in my health too. I really like to garden, but I am able to spend less and less time doing that because gardening makes my skin itch and feel prickly. I also have allergy problems with my nose and throat now that I had never had before I worked on the oil-spill cleanup.[1]

One of the things that has affected my life in a major way is the chemical sensitivity I developed after the oil-spill cleanup. I always end up with a headache if I use hair spray, and I can't use perfume now because it gives me a headache and often makes me feel angry. Before I worked on the oil spill, I could paint my nails and use polish remover. Now I can't stand it when my daughter uses polish remover. I can't use white-out because it makes me feel sick and headachey and my chest starts to tighten. I have to avoid gasoline and diesel. My parents and my sister who worked the spill with me can't use perfume now either, and we all have to be very careful what cleaning products we use.

Looking back, I can't help thinking how ironic it is that my efforts to earn a little money for college working on the oil-spill cleanup would end up causing me so many health problems.

---

[1] Japanese studies have linked chemical exposure to increased allergic reactions to pollen and other allergens. See, for example, *Journal of Allergy and Clinical Immunology* 77 (April 1986): 616-23.

James Handley

EPA Attorney

After spending two years as a trial lawyer at big firms in San Antonio, I was thrilled to be admitted to the Master of Laws program in environmental law at George Washington University in 1987. I had pursued chemical engineering and law degrees as preparation for a career in environmental protection, and the specialized program at GW promised to open doors into my chosen field. My thesis adviser noted my undergraduate degree in chemical engineering and referred me for a work-study program under John Wheeler, an attorney in the EPA's Waste Enforcement Division. John was leading the EPA's legal team on the Love Canal Superfund case.

My first visit to the EPA headquarters in the Waterside Mall in southwest Washington left an indelible impression: the building is one of the most dreary, depressing, and ugly places I've ever set foot in. Wheeler escorted me down winding corridors that were so narrow that two people could barely pass. These hallways were dimly lit by flickering blue fluorescent lights and were punctuated by missing ceiling tiles and stacks of worn-out office equipment, boxes, and other junk. A stale, vaguely chemical odor hung in the air.

Wheeler's dark office was deep in the interior of the building, far from any windows or sources of natural light or fresh air. As I sat in his guest chair, he studied my résumé and said that my chemistry and litigation background would be very useful for the cases in their branch. He was sure they could find plenty of interesting work for me, so we set up my work schedule. A few days later, I reported to the office and began carefully reading and summarizing the chemistry experts' depositions in the Missouri dioxin case. In this notorious case, a waste hauler had accepted "still bottoms" (thick, oily distillation waste) from a chemical plant that made hexachlorophene, an antibacterial ingredient used in soaps. Instead of taking the waste, which contained dioxin, to a permitted facility and paying the required disposal fee, the hauler had simply cracked open the valve on the back of his tank truck and dribbled the oily waste onto the roads in the area, apparently pocketing the disposal fee. His mischief came to light when horses started dying at a stable where he had, for a fee, oiled the dirt paths. The story triggered extensive TV and press coverage, particularly on CBS's "60 Minutes. "

I was eager to apply my chemical engineering course work in organic chemistry, distillation processes, and analytical chemistry to this important environmental enforcement case. Before the semester was over, I had methodically read and summarized a mountain of chemistry depositions and probably knew more about the chemistry aspects of the case (which were key to establishing liability) than anyone else in the government.

As the semester ended, our branch chief asked me if I would be willing to shift to a part-time class schedule at George Washington University the next semester so that I could start working full-time at the EPA. His branch was facing deadlines in the Missouri dioxin case as well as the Love Canal litigation and related cases in the Niagara Falls area. My dream of becoming an environmental protection lawyer and having the privilege of working on some of the key national cases was coming true.

The EPA office where I first worked was generally grim. It was cramped, noisy, and vaguely smoky (the EPA had only recently prohibited smoking in the building). Then in April 1988 we moved to newly renovated offices off a corridor on the other side of the Waterside Mall. Although we were excited to be leaving our ugly old offices and cubicles, my colleagues and I immediately noticed the powerful solvent odor from the new carpet that had been installed the weekend before we unpacked.

At that point, the Love Canal case was busy enough that John Wheeler and I would often work weekends. Every time I entered the building, especially on weekends when the ventilation was not running, I was struck by the pungent "new carpet" smell. Many people complained of headaches and burning eyes. I also felt a burning sensation in my nose and throat and felt so sleepy that I started drinking tea just to stay awake.

Amy Svoboda, another young lawyer in our branch, seemed to be especially hard hit by the polluted air in our building. She sometimes slurred her words, just didn't finish her thoughts, or said things that didn't quite make sense. And I noticed that she seemed more severely affected by the end of the day. She and I agreed to take each other on fresh air breaks two or three times a day to regain our alertness and diminish our symptoms. I was distressed to notice Amy's condition worsening week by week and was also frightened when I gradually realized that I was experiencing similar effects. In addition to my burning eyes and throat, I started to notice that I just couldn't think clearly and sometimes completely forgot what I was doing.

At branch meetings, our health problems became a regular agenda item. We decided to survey all the members of the Waste Enforcement Division about any symptoms they might be experiencing. Some people seemed to be symptom-free, but in general the survey results indicated that there was a very widespread problem. We presented the results to our supervisors, but most of them asked questions that suggested that they didn't take the situation seriously or couldn't do much about it.

The local board of the labor union that represented EPA professionals included several toxicologists and chemists, who became interested in the building-related health problems that various EPA staff members were developing. In the union newsletter, which I helped edit, we published articles about these health problems and suggested that affected staff report to the EPA health unit to register their health complaints.

The union's health and safety representatives reported that the building's ventilation system was providing only five to ten percent fresh air into the building. The rest of the meager flow of air from the ceiling vents was recycled indoor air that included air from several rooms containing large high-speed copy machines that operated nearly continuously, spewing chemical fumes into the air. The building owner claimed it was impossible to open the dampers to allow additional fresh air into the building. Often, I could hear the ventilation blowers shut off in the late afternoon, and I began intercepting the maintenance man who shut the blowers off as he clocked out for the day, which was sometimes as early as 3:30 P.M. When we complained, the EPA management assured us the ventilation would be left on until 7 P.M., the end of the EPA flexible-time workday. But within weeks, the building owner had reverted to turning the blowers off early.

On June 25, 1989, Mark Bradley, M.D., an occupational medicine physician who was the health unit doctor, sent a memo to EPA Administrator William Reilly reporting what he had observed during the six months he had been a consultant at the EPA Health Unit:

> At least 80% of the [approximately 60] individuals who I examined, have bone fide medical problems which I believe are caused by working at the Waterside Mall complex. Fifty to sixty percent had symptoms and physical findings . . . typical of "Tight Building Syndrome" . . . eye and throat irritation, headaches . . . some people were severely affected. Thirty to forty percent . . . had symptoms of airway hyperreactivity . . . a form of occupational asthma. Ten percent of patients had evidence of allergic alveolitis, an inflammatory reaction in the alveoli and bronchioles of the lung resulting from an immune interaction between inhaled organic particles, circulating antibodies and sensitized lymphocites [*sic*]. This condition can be progressive, leading to progressive pulmonary impairment and death. . . . I am certain that . . . I saw only a small fraction of the people . . . potentially adversely affected. . . . There is a major public health situation at this location, and . . . [it] is not being dealt with in a timely, positive and responsible fashion.

The EPA's response to Dr. Bradley (a contract employee) was to immediately terminate his employment.

In one particularly troubling incident, an attorney in the Air Division passed out and was carried out of the building on a stretcher. Everyone was concerned, but there was still no action from management. The EPA professionals' union seemed to be the only organization doing anything about the problem. The union was pressing for removal of what we now called "the toxic carpet," but was meeting resistance from management and also from some staff who preferred carpet to tile floors. Our division managers agreed to remove the carpet only if there was a consensus in favor of doing so. Two attorneys resisted, raising concerns about the noise that a bare floor would engender. Everyone else agreed that a little noise was far less harmful than the toxic fumes that were knocking us all out. Finally, on February 2, 1990, management announced that at the end of the week, the carpet would be removed from rooms in the area where I and most of the Waste Enforcement

Division staff worked. By then, we had been breathing the carpet fumes for almost two years.

A few months later the union got the EPA to agree to have the carpet removed from the rest of the headquarters building. The EPA never admitted a problem, but EPA employees had been featured on several news shows concerning the carpet situation. On CBS's "Street Stories," Ed Bradley had interviewed me and Bill Hirzy, a Ph.D. chemist who later became president of our union. For weeks after the story aired, the union's answering machine was loaded with messages from people all over the country asking for advice about similar health problems caused by new carpet. By this point, it was clear that the carpet that the General Services Administration had procured for the EPA was very low grade. It may even have been off-specification and therefore sold at a discount. For instance, if the chemical reaction to cross-link the polymer in the carpet backing had not been carried out or completed properly, excess monomer (a smaller and lighter molecule) would have remained in the carpet, vaporizing over time and also making the carpet wear out faster.

The Waterside Mall had been constructed to house retail stores and had then been converted into a densely packed government office building. Staff had complained about inadequate ventilation from the beginning of the EPA's occupancy. Installing cheap and probably defective carpet that released solvents into a poorly ventilated building was a formula for a gas chamber.

After the removal of the carpet, many people still experienced indoor air symptoms in Waterside Mall. Their health problems were compounded when in September 1990, several months after the carpet had been removed, contractors began to replace the building's flat asphalt roof. This operation continued over the next several months. Workers on the roof heated tar in caldrons and applied it to the roof. Because the intake vents for the building's ventilation system are also on the roof, the tar fumes got sucked into the vents that supplied our offices.

One day another attorney and I were at a meeting on the fifth floor of the West Tower. From that vantage point, we could see below us the roof of the mall, where the roofing work was being done over our offices. We could see the caldrons of tar with the gray vapor rising a few feet and then curling back down as it was sucked into the building through a nearby air intake. The pungent, sulfurous smell of tar permeated our offices for months. Thick, gray smoke frequently impaired the visibility in the corridors and offices. Inhaling the smoke made my head ache and my chest tighten, as if someone were sitting on me, so it was a struggle to breathe.

After weeks of staff complaints about the roof tar fumes, our deputy division director sent out a memo allowing people to take work home if the fumes made them sick. He also allowed us to bring in air filters. At the union's insistence, the EPA began to allow people who had medical documentation to work at home. It seemed impossible for me to manage to work from home with a team of others all the time, so I only worked at home a few afternoons a week. I often took work outside the building, however, and sat on a bench in a nearby park. Branch meetings were cumbersome; we had to meet outside the building so that the sick people who were working at home, like Amy Svoboda, could join us. We met in adjacent buildings like the public library and Southwest University.

On February 25, 1991, the roof tar fumes were particularly thick. While I was participating in a conference call in my branch chief's office, I lost consciousness. He was stunned and suggested that I take the option of working at home all the time. To make this possible, I needed to start obtaining medical documentation. Up to that point, I had viewed the building air problem as more or less a temporary inconvenience to me, although I could clearly see that others were getting seriously ill.

I often had burning eyes and nasal membranes, a tight feeling in my chest, bouts of fatigue and forgetfulness, headaches, light-headedness, dizziness, "brain fog," a vague achiness throughout my body, and an unquenchable thirst. I could not keep long distance telephone numbers in mind long enough to dial them, so I had to rearrange my desk so I could read the numbers while pressing the phone keys. Another disturbing symptom was a twitching in my eyes and face. All these symptoms except the fatigue, which was becoming constant, seemed to begin soon after I entered the building and then diminish a few hours or a day after I left.

My doctor ordered a spirometry test, which measures the maximum rate and volume of air exhalation and plots it on a graph against time. I blew as hard and fast as I could into a tube, and the machine plotted the results on a graph. We repeated the test the next Monday after I had been away from the office for the weekend. I was surprised to see that the graphs were markedly different. I had exhaled more air and did so much faster after spending the weekend away from the Waterside Mall. My doctor wrote a letter to my supervisor saying that the building appeared to be adversely affecting my health and that if possible I should be allowed to work at home. That letter enabled me to move my office to my house, which was near Capitol Hill.

After the carpet had been removed and the re-roofing completed, the EPA ordered a contractor to perform a study of the indoor air. Air monitors were set up in various parts of the building. During the test, the building's ventilation fans ran faster than we had ever heard them running before. For the first time, we noticed that papers were blowing off people's desks, and the air in the building had never been fresher. Even under those unusually good conditions, the study results showed elevated levels of contamination and documented the fact that many people were experiencing health problems. Unfortunately, no measurements had ever been made while the new carpet and tar fumes were present in the offices. Such measurements would have helped explain the illnesses of hundreds of EPA employees.

Eventually, the sick employees were forced to face the reality that virtually the entire politically appointed management of the EPA was completely indifferent to our plight and unwilling to help us, despite their occasional pronouncements of concern. We were bogged down in a deeply entrenched culture of denial. The EPA management continued to deny and obstruct resolution of the building problems. The chief of the Health and Safety Division even distributed on April 27, 1993, a memo prohibiting the use of air filters in the building. He asserted that they were for home use and had not been shown to work in our office settings, and he also objected to the cost of electricity to operate the filters.

Over the years, the union had learned quite a bit about the carpet and had found that its backing was made with styrene-butadiene latex, which was widely used in the carpet industry. When Bill Hirzy, Ph.D., asked Dr. Rosalind Anderson, a toxicologist, to study samples of the carpet that had been removed from Waterside Mall, she found that even relatively brief exposures to samples of the carpet caused immediate symptoms in mice. Dr. Anderson discovered that the carpet was emitting 4-phenylcyclohexane, a potent neurotoxicant that is apparently an unwanted by-product when latex is polymerized.

Armed with this information, Bill Hirzy and I persuaded Representatives Bernie Sanders and Mike Synar, who chaired the House Oversight Committee for Governmental Affairs, to call a hearing on June 11, 1993, to ask the EPA, the CPSC (Consumer Product Safety Commission), OSHA (Office of Safety and Health Administration), NIOSH (National Institute of Science and Health), and the carpet industry why people were getting sick from carpet and what the agencies were doing about it.

At the hearing that was held on June 11, 1993, union representatives and Dr. Anderson testified. She had videotaped an experiment that showed the effects of the carpet on mice. Dr. Anderson had the mice run down a narrow track under four conditions. First, was the control group that had not been exposed to the carpet. The second group had spent one hour in a vented chamber with the carpet. The third group had spent two hours in the chamber; the fourth group, three hours. The control mice navigated the track easily and quickly. The mice exposed for an hour weaved about somewhat and were visibly slowed down. The mice exposed for two hours didn't all complete the run; some fell off the track. The mice exposed for three hours were comatose or dead.

Bill Hirzy asked me to meet Dr. Anderson at her hotel and take her to dinner the night before the hearing to discuss her testimony. Over dinner, I decided to ask her some questions that I thought might come up at the hearing and were also of keen interest to me. Why, I asked, weren't the people (including me) who had worked in offices with that same carpet for over a year not more visibly affected, or even dead, like the mice? She expected the question but warned me that I might not like the answer. She admitted that she couldn't answer from an empirical point of view, but she pointed out that humans have a lot more redundancy in their brains than mice do. She suggested that our brains had been harmed in the same way that the mice brains were, but that because our brains are larger, they could reroute the signals and were able to cope with higher doses for longer times. The damage was like a series of small strokes, she said. Small injuries that add up. And if any of us were ever hit on the head or had a stroke or got Parkinson's or Alzheimer's, we might have fewer "spare parts" to compensate. That news didn't make my dinner go down well, but it made sense. It meant that in terms of brain function, I and my colleagues were effectively driving with a flat tire.

The next day's congressional hearing was just beautiful. The room was crowded with press and EPA staff wearing buttons that said "Protect the Environment of EPA Employees." After Dr. Anderson explained her research and showed her video to the committee, the reaction was stunned silence. The EPA management offered excuses, but primarily maintained that carpet toxicity wasn't something EPA could address. The Consumer Products Safety Commission looked ridiculous; its representative said there wasn't enough scientific certainty to take action yet. The carpet industry didn't admit any health problems but proposed to attach warning labels to carpet suggesting that sensitive people air new carpet out for a while and watch for symptoms. I'm not aware of any congressional, EPA, or CPSC action that followed that hearing, but I noticed that over the succeeding years carpet with styrene-butadiene backing seemed to have disappeared from the stores.

*   *   *   *   *

I was eventually able to transfer to the Toxics and Pesticides Enforcement Division, which was moving out of Waterside Mall to the Ariel Rios Federal Building. I requested and was assigned to an office with an operable window to accommodate my chemical sensitivity, and for about five years, I was able to work there productively with few reactions to airborne contaminants. In 2000, however, after coping with sporadic health problems in the Rios Building, my health began to decline once again when renovations were started in nearby areas that included sanding the floors and refinishing them with polyurethane. At that point, having been made sick twice before by chemical exposures, I decided to get a thorough medical evaluation to document my symptoms and injury. I consulted with a widely published expert on chemical brain injury, Dr. Kaye Kilburn at the University of Southern California. His examination included four hours of tests, and he found strong evidence of chemical brain injury. After considering my situation carefully, I submitted the required documentation to seek early retirement. The materials I submitted included not only Dr. Kilburn's report but also observations by my branch chief about my low energy level when I was exposed to chemicals and specifics about how I had become disoriented and ill after exposures to diesel exhaust during a business trip with him. Within a few months, the Office of Personnel Management offered me early retirement at a small fraction of my salary.

While I was fearful about my financial future, I knew that my symptoms were progressing and I couldn't count on getting another chance like that, so I left the EPA at the end of November 2000. It was an anguishing decision to relinquish my career, which was a very important part of my identity, but my dream job had become a nightmare. I had worked at the forefront of environmental issues that I consider vital to the future of my country, but I had also found repeatedly that the agency charged with environmental protection was unwilling or unable to protect its own employees and was also stunningly ineffectual at protecting the public or the larger environment.

Wanda Phillips

FEMA Trailer Exposure

The field in front of my house in Purvis, Mississipi, used to be the home of beautiful long-horned steers that grazed peacefully on the thick green grass. The cows would lift their heads and low softly when my grandchildren would climb on the fence and wave their hands excitedly at them. My husband and I used to sit on the breezeway of our porch and watch the cows grazing, and we thanked God for blessing us with the opportunity to live in such a beautiful home in the country. Now the grass on that field has been brutally scraped off. Truckloads of crushed rock have been brought in to make roadways and driveways; the remainder of the field is now bare dirt that blows wildly across the area when the wind rises. The beautiful long-horned steers have been replaced by white elephants–FEMA trailers–brought in by the federal government. The cows' soft lowing has been replaced by the piercing, chirping warnings given off by the dying batteries of trailer alarms. FEMA, a federal agency I had never heard of before Hurricane Katrina, has become a new way of life for my family.

All pretense of privacy is gone; it's been replaced by guards with guns, ever watchful for movement from any direction. The guards nod with an impersonal nod and sometimes ask who won what game when we go to retrieve the daily newspaper. When we look out the window or walk out onto the porch or into the yard, the eyes of bored security guards are there watching us. Also gone with our privacy is the lost health that we enjoyed without realizing what we had until it was gone.

I will never forget the tremendous excitement I felt when I witnessed Katrina's outrageous display of force. Our huge trees fell slowly as the wind caught their branches like umbrellas and lifted them, pulling their roots from the ground in slow motion and leaving them exposed to the rain that fell in sheets. It sounded like trains and eighteen wheelers were tearing down the highway in front of our house and through the woods behind the house.

But the regret at the loss of our trees and the damage to our house is nothing compared to the hurt, anger, and pain that I have and am experiencing from the stonewalling of the federal government as it turns a blind eye to the problems that my family is experiencing. Unfortunately, the federal government decided that the best place to set up a huge operation to help Hurricane Katrina victims was right across the road from our house. In the course of setting up their operation, they blocked the road with traffic. The FEMA trailers arrived at the cow pasture pulled by what looked to us like grannies and young boys not old enough for the job. It appeared that every unemployed person had jumped on the bandwagon to try to make a fast big buck. We even heard of people quitting their jobs to pull FEMA trailers. We watched in amazement at the strange assortment of people pulling the trailers into the new staging facility. Most of the drivers appeared to be inexperienced and new to this type of work.

In the first stages of setting up camp, FEMA installed a garbage dumpster and a long row of porta potties right across the street from my home. For over eighteen months, we could see these porta potties and dumpster from our kitchen and we could smell them from our dining room table. For over eighteen months, our house was lit up inside at night like a Christmas tree. As we lay in bed, we could feel the rumbling of the generators that ran all night long to power the floodlights that lit up the staging facility across the road. During the day, multiple smaller generators ran. Even now dust fills my house from the raw exposed earth across the road from my house. We can hear cell phones ringing and the garbled voices of people laughing and talking as they go about FEMA business. We listen to people shouting to make themselves heard above the generators and the slamming of the porta-potty doors. A business of this magnitude leaves a big footprint.

All my life I have worked hard. I have struggled and gone to school with holes in my shoes and my toes exposed, so ashamed that I finally quit school after the ninth grade. I have cooked on a wood stove and milked a cow to provide my children with milk. I grew up poor enough that at times we did not have running water and toted water from a spring that we dug under the hill to get water to drink and to use to wash our clothes in the bathtub. Many times we bathed in the evenings in the Escatawpa River or took a cold sponge bath in front of a small heater. I have worked hard and long to arrive to where I am now. I have a new life where I never go to bed hungry and don't have to survive on deer meat and field peas. I don't have to beg the power man not to turn off

my power. Now in the peak of my life when my children are grown and
have moved out and I am still young enough and financially able to ride
my motorcycle on long motorcycle trips, skydive, or go hiking in the
mountains, it's hard to do those things I love because I am sick.

My health problems started with a dripping nose and coughing that
I first attributed to allergies. I had been diagnosed with asthma and
allergies before FEMA moved in across the road and started sharing my
life, but allergy shots had helped me. It had been years since I had any
problems with allergies, and even though my doctor said I had asthma
I couldn't tell it. After FEMA moved in, I developed a cough that still
bothers me. I was rechecked for allergies, and my allergies came back
insignificant, so that was not the problem. My husband developed
chronic sinus drainage that became so serious that he had to have
surgery. Before FEMA moved in across the road, he had sleep apnea.
After they moved in, he developed a new and horrifying symptom in his
sleep that he had never had before. His snoring and occasional noises at
night changed to a terrifying strangling that he would describe as
drowning in his sleep. Then he started having this strangulation feeling
when he was just sitting in his recliner. His doctor performed surgery to
trim back his elongated pallet and straighten his deviated septum; he
also removed his uvula. None of my husband's problems were alleviated
by this procedure; the only thing that happened is that now he chokes
and vomits easily.

I have always thought that my husband's problem was related to the
FEMA operation across the road. I can still remember the expression of
shock on his face when I told him we needed to move away from this.
Shock and disbelief. All he said was, "and go where?"

It was not easy to persuade my husband that we needed to move, but
by this point I had decided that my health was more important than
anything else and that I would move without him if necessary. I did a
hardship withdrawal from my 401(k) and started developing a raw piece
of property that I owned in my hometown of Richton, Mississippi, about
forty-five minutes from our home in Purvis. The development process
on my land in Richton was slow going, however, because all the contractors and equipment operators in the area were busy doing hurricane
repairs. About the same time that I was at last able to get the utilities
installed at my property in Richton and to get my hurricane repairs done
at my home in Purvis, FEMA started auctioning off the used trailers that

were being returned to the staging facility across from us by hurricane survivors who were blessed enough to escape them. I told my husband that we might as well buy one so that I could live in it on my land in Richton until the FEMA operation across from us shut down.

We looked at hundreds of trailers, but only a few passed our inspection sufficiently that we were willing to bid on them. Lots of the trailers were warped and twisted. The floors buckled up in the center, the walls were leaning, the windows were busted out, and mold was growing in and on them. Some had bullet holes in them, and some of the trailers had undergone fire damage. A guard told me that some people in New Orleans had used the trailers to make crystal meth and they had exploded and burned. My husband and I thought that one reason there were so many problems with the trailers was that FEMA was using inexperienced people to pull them, set them up, and do maintenance on them. Who ever heard of putting an RV on blocks? I can just imagine what putting the trailers on blocks did to the integrity of the structures.

The condition of the trailers was terrible. The pet odors in some were so awful you would gag when you went in the door. Finally, I was able to win the bid on a small FEMA spec trailer; the structure looked intact and it had a strong "new" smell to it.

What I didn't know at that time was that the incredible new smell in my new FEMA trailer was in fact caused by formaldehyde. In time, I would learn more about formaldehyde than I would ever want to know. I have recently had a chemical testing company test the formaldehyde levels in my FEMA trailer, and the results were high. I didn't know that, however, when I moved into my new trailer and my husband soon grudgingly followed me. Within the next months, we spent most of our time in the FEMA trailer. My pregnant daughter and her two daughters were with us as well. We spent the evenings cleaning up hurricane damage on the property and would fall exhausted into bed at night. We did not cook in the trailer or do much of anything but sleep in it because it was so small. We went by our home in Purvis from time to time in the evening so that people wouldn't realize we were no longer living there.

Finally, my husband decided to go back home to Purvis to live because he was worried that with all the increased traffic in front of our house it might be robbed. In addition, he had trouble sleeping in the trailer, which was also a problem for me, even though I had bought an expensive mattress to use in it. Later we learned that insomnia can be a symptom of formaldehyde exposure. At any rate, the longer I stayed in the trailer, the sicker I became. The stress of the cramped quarters and the girls climbing up and down the bunk beds like monkeys made me decide that if I was going to be sick wherever I was, I might as well be sick in the comfort of our big brick house, so we all went back to Purvis. By this time, however, it had ceased to feel like my home; it had become just the house where I dwelled.

Even before the *Hattiesburg American* ran the first article about formaldehyde in the FEMA trailers, we had noticed that we could smell the trailers across the road when we sat on our front porch. I had also begun to lose my voice when I sat outside in the evenings. It is now common for me to lose my voice at the slightest provocation. My doctor had me tested for everything that he could think of that would make you lose your voice or be hoarse, and everything has come back fine. He has told me that the only thing he can do is treat my symptoms. I quit going outside and stayed in the house all the time.

My whole life changed because of the FEMA trailers because I am now sensitive to lots of different chemicals. I have had to quit using candles and plug-in air fresheners. Many of the cleaners that I formerly used now irritate my sinuses and will start a storm of coughing and sinus drainage. The sinus drainage makes the skin on the top of my soft pallet feel like it has been scraped with a wire brush. I have had to give up coloring my hair because the dye started giving me bad headaches and made me feel dizzy and nauseated. I also had to quit wearing makeup because when I put on eye makeup, my eyes would water and soon all the makeup would be gone. My husband bought me a new four-door Jeep for Valentines Day, but I don't drive it because the new smell makes me cough and my nose run. There have been times that I have coughed until I have had to wrap my arms around my ribs because it felt like my ribs were going to break. Bronchitis and horrifying green drainage from my nose has become an everyday occurrence.

Tests of the formaldehyde level in the outside ambient air in front of our house have shown levels twice the amount considered safe for year-round living conditions. Scientists have said that formaldehyde is a carcinogen. Cancer is something that I have dealt with before. After a couple of surgeries I have been cancer free for over twelve years, but the fear of it is still with me, intensified by my knowledge that there are carcinogenic levels of formaldehyde in my front yard.

I worry especially about my youngest granddaughter because my daughter had such difficulty carrying her. By the time she was three-months-old, my granddaughter had had a couple of spells where she quit breathing and her legs from the knees down turned blue. In my research, I have found that there are documented cases of birth defects caused by exposure to formaldehyde in the first trimester of pregnancy. My daughter lived with me for three or four days every week during her pregnancy and still continues to stay with me. She and my grand-daughters also stayed with me in our FEMA trailer. My daughter had recurrent labor for weeks before her daughter was born. She took medications for the problem and was admitted to the hospital on more than one occasion to stop her from giving birth too early. Even then she delivered her baby early.

My son-in-law coughs and spits and blows his nose nonstop when he is at my house. I can see my family having the same problems that I have experienced with the headaches and earaches and other symptoms, but at a lower rate. Everybody's immune system is different, but apparently no one is immune to the effects of continuous toxins. I had hoped that one day FEMA would leave and we could get well, but I have been told that they are here to stay. I have also learned that once a large chemical exposure makes you develop a sensitivity to all sorts of other chemicals, you have a disability that will probably affect you for the rest of your life. I pray that my family and I will not be permanently damaged by our formaldehyde exposure.

I am making arrangements to move again, away from my home and the slumbering white elephants across the street. Of course, it won't be easy to sell our present house, given the monstrous trailer site across the road. I get so tired of everyone telling us that our home has lost its value and that we will never be able to sell it. That's just one more way that FEMA has had a huge impact on my life.

If the trailer site isn't shut down, then my last resort is to move to my property in Richton, Mississippi, and build a home there. I have now purchased a twenty-four-year-old trailer that I can put on my land in Richton while I'm waiting to build a house. The only reason I haven't started to build a new house yet is that now the federal government wants to expand the Strategic Petroleum Reserve and has announced that a new SPR facility will be located in Richton, Mississippi, as part of the expansion project. The government wants to clean out the salt domes in Richton and store millions of gallons of petroleum two and a half miles across the swamp from my property. Reports I have read say that about six square miles of the salt area appears suitable for cavern development. Does this mean that there will be huge amounts of petroleum below my land? I no longer trust our government to look out for my health and welfare, so I'm at a loss to know whether to build a house there or not.

Sfc. Terry Dillhyon

Gulf War Veteran

I was in the Marine Corps from 1960 to 1966. When I left the Corps, I got a job with a major railroad company as a steel worker building rail cars. I started a family and earned a college degree by attending classes at night while I worked for the railroad.

In November 1990, I was activated with my Army National Guard unit and sent to the Persian Gulf. I served both as a medic and as an intelligence NCO. Prior to the Gulf War, I was in perfect health and in great physical condition. Now I'm in a wheelchair.

I spent that Christmas Eve of 1990 in an unforgettable sandstorm that some said was one of the worst sandstorms that had ever been recorded in Saudi Arabia. The storm hit on Christmas Eve, when we had just been trying to put together a makeshift Christmas tree using chemical lights—those plastic straws that glow in the dark. Anyway, the wind quickly became so strong that everyone inside our tent was ordered to hold the sides of the tent so it wouldn't blow away. The strength of the wind blew fine sand right through the canvas, so we had to put our ponchos in front of our faces to keep from being choked by the dust. It was a sandstorm and a Christmas Eve that none of us who had arrived in the Persian Gulf early will ever forget.

One of my jobs as a medic was to pass out malaria pills to the troops in our unit every day. There were lots of mosquitoes around, so malaria was a real threat. As a result, we used a lot of DEET. We had two kinds of government issue—a cream to put on our skin and spray cans containing what you might call industrial strength DEET. We weren't supposed to spray the stronger version in confined spaces, but lots of soldiers used it when they ran out of the cream, which was pretty often. They would spray it on their skin and uniforms while they were inside the tent. Some troops even wore flea collars around their wrists and ankles.

We were stationed in Ryad in Saudi Arabia for much of the Gulf War. There were lots of SCUD attacks on Ryad. Almost every time there was a SCUD attack, our chemical alarms would go off, but higher authorities claimed the instruments were all defective and were giving us false alarms.

Like almost everyone else in the Gulf War, I had to take the pyridostigmine bromide pills. About three days after I started taking them, I developed a stomach ache and nausea. I saw some other people throw up and even saw some people throw up blood. Women had a worse reaction than men. The pills didn't seem to bother some people at all, however.

When we returned to the United States, we received the most minimal physical you could ever give to servicemen returning from war. I went back to work with the railroad but continued to serve in the Army National Guard. After returning to work, I started having problems that I had never had before. The automatic air freshener dispenser in our office was making me sick, as were paint and diesel fumes. I started having panic attacks, and I was having problems concentrating on my work and other activities. I no longer could climb to the top of railroad cars. One morning I had a terrible headache, a stiff neck, and a very high fever. I was rushed to the emergency room, where they did a spinal tap. The doctor did not find anything, but he treated me for spinal meningitis.

Everything seemed to get worse from that point on. I was falling down at work for no good reason. In January 1993, I could not pass the Army Physical Fitness Test and had to retire from the Army National Guard. That year I started using a cane because my right ankle and leg just kept giving way as I walked.

After I left the National Guard, I went to the VA hospital in my area and signed up for the Gulf War Registry and took the Gulf War Veterans' Physical. I was placed in the hospital for one week. My condition got worse, and in March 1993, I was sent to the VA hospital in Washington, D.C., for more tests. I was only supposed to stay in the hospital for seven to ten days, but they kept me there for six weeks.

My discharge summary was panic disorder, degenerative joint disease, severe high frequency hearing lost in right ear, allergic rhinitis, emphysema, high cholesterol, chronic fatigue syndrome, possible multiple chemical sensitivity, mild patchy sensory neuropathy of distal nerve segments, and multifocal motor neuropathy with conduction blocks of the ulnar and radial nerves of both arms. The doctors stated regarding all the above medical problems: "etiology unknown." The doctor who told me I had multiple chemical sensitivity said he wasn't allowed to write that in the diagnosis—he could only say "possible multiple chemical sensitivity."

In 1994, I had to start using two canes, and that worked for about six months. If I happened to smell something like gasoline or perfume, however, it would affect my coordination and I would fall down. Finally, the Veterans Administration gave me a wheelchair, and a couple of years ago they even gave me an electric one because I have a lot of nerve damage in my arms. I can't complain about the medical care the VA has given me. They have paid for my medications and hospitalizations, even though they claim my problems are not service-connected.

When I returned home from the VA hospital in Washington, the railroad company would not let me return to work and retired me on disability. I could not understand what was going on because I had always been very healthy before I went to the Gulf War. I contacted my VA representative to file a claim for service connected disability, but I have not received anything from the VA Disability Board. Other vets who worked right beside me in the Gulf War have received disability compensation for diagnoses like fibromyalgia and chronic fatigue syndrome, but I don't know of anyone who has been given a disability award for MCS.

When I went to a civilian doctor in connection with my application to obtain Medicare coverage from the Social Security Administration, I happened to mention that I had MCS. He went ballistic and said, "So you're one of those people. Let me tell you what, you just lost all your credibility with me." He turned in a negative report to the Social Security board, which then denied me Medicare coverage. I have, however, been on Social Security disability payments since 1995.

I have had several other medical problems in the past eight years. I have skin rashes and sores, stomach problems, and chronic pain. Before the Gulf War, I would very seldom take an aspirin or any other kind of medication. I worked very hard all the time and never took time off from work because of illness. Now I take twenty-five pills a day. I am no longer permitted to drive, and I am having a very hard time adjusting to that.

Before the war, I had been stung by bees on several occasions and never had a bad reaction. Now bee stings bring on anaphylactic shock. One time when I was stung and my wife was rushing me to the hospital, our route was blocked by a passing train. She quickly whipped the car around and tried another route, only to find that a truck full of watermelons had overturned and blocked that road. She was in a panic by that time because my swelling was increasing and my throat was closing off so that I could barely breathe. Fortunately, by the time we returned to the first road, the train had passed. When we got to the emergency room and my wife ran inside to get help taking me in, a nurse came rushing out and had me drop my pants right there in the parking lot so she could give me the shot.

My problems with chemical sensitivity began right after the Gulf War. I still cannot pump gas or diesel fuel; my wife pumps it while I sit in the car or truck with the windows rolled up. The ink smell on a fresh newspaper really bothers me. I have to watch what type of shampoo I use or I will break out in a bad rash. Some perfumes also give me a bad reaction. Just last week I started to read a magazine, and it turned out it had a perfume strip in it. I got immediately nauseated and got a headache; I felt so sick I had to go to bed. The next morning I was still nauseated and was wheezing, so I had to go to the hospital. They kept me there a couple of days. I had another bad reaction to perfume when I went to my grandson's kindergarten graduation. I had to be carried out of the building because someone was wearing a perfume that was so strong that I could not breathe and got very sick.

It is very hard living with multiple chemical sensitivity because there are so many chemicals that can make you really sick very fast. To me, MCS is not a joke and should not be taken lightly. It's had a terrible effect on my life.

Rachel Hughes

9/11 Exposure

After the terrorist attacks on the World Trade Center, I wanted to do something to help, so on September 12, I volunteered to help unload trucks and pass out sandwiches and water to rescue workers. At the time, I was only thirty-five and was in excellent health. I didn't realize that my volunteer work at Ground Zero might jeopardize my health for the rest of my life.

Within days of the 9/11 attacks, I had a fever and a constant headache; I was also vomiting and feeling dizzy. A bad cough made it hard for me to sleep. I was also having trouble breathing and had considerable chest pain and tightness. One of my worst problems was that large, unsightly sores started erupting on my scalp, face, neck, arms, and back.

About a week after 9/11, I returned to work at my office, which was located about eight blocks north of the Trade Towers. In my director's job in a multimedia company, I managed hundreds of employees and projects. When we returned to work, there was still thick dust all over our office, so we had to help clean our work spaces ourselves. I wore a surgical mask to work for several weeks because the air smelled horrible and was so thick with dust that it was hard to breathe, despite the assurances from the head of the EPA that the air was safe to breathe. I hoped the mask would help lessen my cough, but it didn't. Even three months later the smoke in the area still made my eyes sting. Despite all the smoke and dust and fumes, I continued to work full-time in Lower Manhattan until I was laid off in December 2001 because of the negative effect 9/11 had on business.

My health problems related to the 9/11 toxic exposures have steadily worsened. I frequently have pneumonia or bronchitis, and this can mean that I have to rest in bed and not work for months at a time. Even then I feel only slightly better. In the seven years since 9/11, I have not had one day when I have felt healthy and energetic the way I used to feel. Daily headaches are a problem, and I continue to have constant chest pain, pressure, and shortness of breath with the slightest exertion. My diagnoses include lung scarring. A night cough that is only alleviated by sitting upright makes sleeping extremely difficult. For months at a time, I run low grade fevers and have swollen, painful lymph glands in my neck and other areas. I have muscle and joint pain, prickly numbness in my legs and arms and across my back, and fatigue so intense that it makes it difficult to even take a shower without needing to rest afterward. Simple household tasks like doing the laundry or grocery shopping are exhausting.

During the first couple of years of my 9/11-related illness, I was misdiagnosed by my doctor, who told me that all these symptoms were the result of stress. One doctor I consulted told me I was becoming a hypochondriac. For a few years, I did what those doctors said. I ignored my symptoms and attempted to work. I also pushed myself at the gym to do yoga as I had done before 9/11. But things just worsened with this exercise regimen, and I was having trouble making it through a day.

My situation during this time was particularly difficult because my doctor was not running any tests or diagnosing me with anything other than stress. Hence for a few years I kept my symptoms and illness a secret from most of my friends, family, and co-workers. I began to do less and less, however, because I didn't feel like being around people when I was feeling ill and couldn't explain to them what was going on. Finally, three years after 9/11, I began telling people that I had been sick and had been pretending earlier that I was going to work when I was too sick to leave my home and had to spend much of the day in bed. Because I have not been able to work for years, I have now spent all my savings, have had to sell my car and my home, and can no longer afford to rent my painting studio. Now I'm $100,000 in debt to family and friends and facing bankruptcy because of medical bills.

By the spring of 2004, I realized I needed to find a doctor who had experience dealing with patients with my range of symptoms so that I could find out what was causing them. I was diagnosed with chronic fatigue syndrome and fibromyalgia in 2004. By early 2005, physicians in the Mount Sinai WTC Medical Monitoring Program diagnosed me as having immune system dysfunction, chemical asthma, gastrointestinal disorders and sinusitis. In addition, tests by other doctors showed that my thyroid and adrenal glands were not working right and that I have high levels of mercury, lead, and other toxic chemicals in my body.

Chemical sensitivity became a significant problem for me after my exposure to 9/11 toxins. Since that point, I have become sensitive to all types of chemical fumes that never gave me any problems before. I have had to stop wearing perfume and start using unscented body lotion and shampoo. The chemicals like ammonia or solvents that they use to clean the elevator or halls in my building make it difficult for me to breathe and sometimes give me a migraine. I actually try to hold my breath in the elevator because the cleaning products affect me so strongly.

I have always been a dedicated artist, but I can't paint right now because I'm too sensitive to the paint, even water-based paint. I'm too sensitive to markers to use them for illustration and drawing. The room in my apartment where I used to do art work after I could no longer afford to rent my art studio has turned into a medical billing station containing files of medical and insurance records.

In September 2004, I did a five-week round of chelation therapy for the metals poisoning, but it did not work as promised. In December 2004, I ended up in the hospital twice because of repeated fainting spells, trouble breathing, and severe exhaustion. I was told I had low blood pressure and was put on oxygen. Later I found out that my adrenal glands were so low functioning that my blood pressure had dropped to 80/40; it was normally 120/80. I was told the chelation treatments would get me back to normal. Instead, I felt worse because of complications with my weakened immune system, kidneys, and liver.

Pulmonary tests in the official WTC monitoring program at Mount Sinai Hospital in NYC have shown that my lungs are functioning at thirty percent below normal capacity. If I breathe too deep, I get a pinching pain in my chest. Other symptoms that no doctor has been able to explain are that my teeth and gums hurt a lot, my eyes hurt, and I still have severe eruptions of sores over my scalp, neck, back, shoulders, and face. In January 2006, I had forty percent of my hair fall out in clumps because of a prescription drug interaction.

Anyone who has met me since my exposure to the 9/11 toxic dust and fumes has only gotten a glimpse of who I am. I hope that I can someday work at my job again and return to volunteering as a teaching artist working with kids in art education programs in the New York City schools. The ''real me'' is not here right now because the ''real me'' is someone with energy and the ability to sleep well and work full-time. The "real me" loved to go to art galleries, attend jazz concerts and the theater; the "real me" enjoyed hitting the gym five days a week, doing daily yoga, spending time with friends and visiting family. I hope my good health will return so I can once more engage in all the things I loved in life.

Victoria Savini

Accountant

In October of 2001, the Hart Senate Office Building was contaminated by mail containing anthrax spores that was sent to two senators. During this time, I was working as an Accounts Payable Specialist in the Disbursing Office. Of course, the building was quickly shut down, and three weeks later we moved to offices in the Postal Square Building.

Since all the mail was potentially tainted, an irradiation process was begun to kill any spores that could be contained in envelopes in the future. This resulted in "over cooking," which made the paper turn to a yellow/brown color and made the pages of letters stick together. The fumes that remained from the process were enough to cause my eyes to water at times.

When I began getting sick that fall, the first thing I noticed was that my hands began to swell and become very painful. I started to think I was getting arthritis or something, however, so I didn't make a connection to the irradiated mail.

In January of 2002, we moved back into the Hart Building. The cleanup for any possible anthrax spores had been completed, and the whole building smelled like chlorine in a swimming pool. Upon returning to the Hart, I began having headaches and severe joint pain. My wrists were hurting so badly I couldn't even lay my hands flat on a table or put any pressure on them at all. When I went to my doctor, I asked him if I might have carpal tunnel syndrome. But since I had problems with my knees and hips and even my toe joints, he thought it might be rheumatoid arthritis, so he sent me to a rheumatologist. My hands at this point were very swollen, and I was missing work here and there because some days I couldn't close my hands to button my clothing and get dressed.

After a thorough examination and x-rays, the rheumatologist told me that she didn't know what was wrong with me but it wasn't rheumatoid arthritis. I returned to work in pain and just kept taking over-the-counter pain medications.

On March 27, 2002, I was working on vouchers and breathed in some unusual fumes from the paper. I felt an odd sensation in my nostrils and then in my throat. I began coughing, and within minutes I completely lost my voice and began having difficulty breathing. I went to the Hart Health Unit, where I was put on oxygen and the paramedics came in along with the Senate's attending physician. They couldn't figure out what had happened and treated me as if it were asthma. The doctor gave me an inhaler to use, and the nurse on duty advised me not to return to work because if there was something in the office causing this reaction, it would happen again.

The next day I visited an emergency care doctor who prescribed Prednisone, Volmax, and two additional inhalers. He also administered a breathing treatment to alleviate any potential restriction in my lungs or throat. At this point I began working closely with workers' compensation. The woman there was extremely helpful to me. She understood how sick I was and told me that there were other people suffering the way I was.

On April 1, 2002, I returned to work after a few days absence. I began coughing within minutes of coming into my office cubicle, and once again I lost my voice. Despite this reaction, I struggled through the day, hoping my coughing fit would cease. That never happened.

On the following morning, the coughing began again immediately after I entered the office. My supervisor told me to go get something to drink, and he thoroughly cleaned and wiped down my workspace from top to bottom. Despite his best efforts, this did not help, and I ended up being sent home by the nurse again. This scenario continued for the coming days. I would report to work, get sick, and then be ordered home by the nurse. During this time, my headaches began to worsen, as well as my joint pain, voice loss, nausea, memory loss, and acid reflux.

On April 7, 2002, the disbursing office decided to move me into another room with a different ventilation system. We were all hoping that would be the "fix" to my dilemma. What no one thought about was that the room they put me in was piled with boxes of irradiated paper. I experienced constant coughing and discomfort in that room, the only difference being that I began coughing even before I started working with the vouchers. No wonder, with all the irradiated paper that was stored in that room.

During this period, I saw two internists; an allergist; an ear, nose, and throat specialist; and a gastroenterologist for my acid reflux. I was tested twice for allergies, and in both instances, the results showed that I was not allergic to any of the common substances that could bring about the kind of reaction that I had been experiencing. The gastroenterologist performed an endoscopy and found that my esophagus had been burned. He said I was fluxing but showed no signs of acid reflux disease and that chemical exposure should be explored. All the doctors concluded the same thing: some type of irritant in the Hart Building was affecting me and I would probably have to eventually leave my job.

Since the experiment of moving me to another room in the Hart Building had not worked, my supervisor decided that I should try working on the vouchers in a room in the Capitol Building to see if I could tolerate working with the vouchers in a different building. But within half an hour of working with the vouchers in this new space, I was coughing and getting a raspy throat. By the time an hour had passed, I had no voice at all and I was feeling nauseated and shaky. I called my doctor's office, and he said I should not to leave the building because I might pass out. He told me to see the attending physician on Capitol Hill, but the only thing that doctor told me was to avoid whatever was causing these episodes. So I gathered up the vouchers and returned to the Hart Building. As I was walking back, I realized that the vouchers were not making me cough even though I was holding them. I realized then that it was handling the irradiated paper in an enclosed environment that was the cause of these episodes and the other symptoms I was experiencing only while at work.

I reported my observations to Human Resources and the Financial Clerk of the Senate, telling them that I probably could handle irradiated paper as long as I was near a window or somewhere with proper ventilation. My walk back to the Hart Building while I was holding those vouchers and not coughing seemed to prove it. I asked to be allowed to work outside as an experiment to see if my theory was correct but was told I couldn't. I then asked once again to be moved to a place with proper ventilation, but the Financial Clerk of the Senate refused my request, saying, "I'll never allow it." When I asked why, he said that if he did it for me, he would have to do it for anyone else in the office who complained, so he would never allow it to happen.

Human Resources in the meantime seemed to be trying to make a case against me. They sent e-mails to my supervisor asking him how many minutes a day I was away from my desk. I knew that they could only let me go if I didn't carry my work load, so it was obvious what was happening. I was facing either being fired or being forced to resign. When I went to workers' compensation for help, I found that my case had been reassigned to a new caseworker who was inexperienced and the original caseworker had been instructed not to speak with me. I knew this was because Human Resources realized she was giving me information that they didn't want me to have.

When I told the new caseworker that I was worried about losing my job because I had two kids in college and my job covered their costs, she said, "What makes you different than anyone else? Just take out loans like the rest of us do." It was clear she was not in my corner and I was basically on my own.

At this time, I was surfing the Internet to find out anything I could about sick building syndrome and irradiated paper. In my search, I found out about a chemical sensitivity conference being held in a Washington suburb, which I quickly registered for and attended. There I met a toxicologist who specializes in chemically induced illnesses and explained to her what was happening to me. She said, "You must leave your job before you get any worse, or it could be too late." Since my voice was still disappearing at work and my other symptoms were getting worse, I realized she was right and I handed in my resignation. I later found out that several unpaid interns had been experiencing the same breathing problems. Since they were unpaid, they just decided to leave rather than fight. I know I was not the only one having problems with the irradiated paper, although the Senate contended that I was.

A year later I saw a news report that described the symptoms being experienced by the people who had been taking antibiotics because they had been exposed to anthrax spores. They had the same symptoms I had but were blaming it on the antibiotics. Since I did not test positive for anthrax exposure, I never took the antibiotic that was offered to me, yet I had the same symptoms as the people who had taken the antibiotics. That's why I believe that it was a combination of the irradiated mail and the fumigation of the Hart Building that was causing these problems.

To this day, I remain hypersensitive to certain substances. I can't even go near a store aisle containing fertilizer or pesticides. Things like perfume or construction odors cause me to develop throat irritation and to cough and lose my voice. Even the smell that is emitted from my car air conditioner and car heater sets me off. The fumes from the fuel on an airplane produce the same problem. I used to be able to fly without any problem, but now I cough and get a raspy voice while on a trip. I never know when some exposure will cause me to start coughing and lose my voice. My hope is that one day the Senate will realize what happened and either stop irradiating the mail or get proper ventilation in these enclosed offices.

When I was hired for my new job at the Woodrow Wilson International Center for Scholars, they made sure I had whatever accommodations they could manage. They changed the post office that their mail went through before I ever got there because some of their other employees were having problems too.

The accommodations they implemented to make it possible for me to work included the following:

1) If anything irradiated made it through to the office, it would be photocopied for me so I wouldn't have to touch the original.

2) One day there was a construction project going on in the building, and immediately after I arrived at my office, my throat closed up, I started coughing, and I lost my voice. My supervisors called a cleaning crew immediately and allowed me to go outside until all the dust from the sheet-rock was cleaned up.

3) Management also gave me a large air filter to keep in my office, which works very well.

4) I always have fair warning if carpets are going to be replaced or special cleaning products are going to be used. My boss will stop by my office and tell me to close the door. If I have any breathing problems, I'm allowed to just go outside without telling anyone because my boss doesn't want me to feel sick.

5) It is understood that if there is a prolonged construction project that affects me adversely, they will provide me with a laptop to work from home.

The most important thing of all is that my superiors believed me when I said I had a problem with certain chemical exposures. They were willing to work with me in any way they could to enable me to continue working. This I consider to be the biggest accommodation any employer could give.

Because of these simple accommodations that my employer provides, I am able to keep working. It's so important for other employers, including the federal government, to realize that people like me can be extremely productive in a job if the employer is willing to do some simple things that allow us to continue working instead of treating us as though we are the ones at fault.

The Potter Brothers

Exxon Valdez Cleanup Workers

The Potter brothers all worked together to clean up the oil-soaked beaches of Prince William Sound, with quite different effects upon their health.

Roger Potter

I heard about the oil spill on the radio at 5 or 6 A.M. on the morning it occurred. My brothers and I thought right away that there might be a job opportunity here. We were union members and hadn't had much work since we had helped build the pipeline up at Prudhoe Bay. After the pipeline was built, the company preferred to hire non-union labor. We had been hunting around for work for years, doing what we could to keep body and soul together. We even cut wood for two years. Our union scale pay for construction work was $23 or $24 an hour, but we were offered only about $17 an hour on the oil spill cleanup. At least we knew we would get lots of overtime; one week I worked 109 hours.

We got our dispatches to report to work on May 5, so we drove down to Valdez, where there was still four feet of snow on the ground. After we arrived, we were sent to an indoctrination session at the Civic Center. There the speakers told us they were unsure what the effect of the 180-odd compounds in the oil would be because they had not all been tested. They said most of the stuff had no Material Safety Data Sheets to let us know how the chemicals might affect us. They told us it was kind of a crap shoot what the long-term or short-term effects would be. A lot of us were looking at each other when we heard that. As I recall, it was just one three- or four-hour session that we had to attend before we started working on the oil-spill cleanup.

My brothers and I were assigned to a berthing vessel called the *Fort McHenry*, where we lived with twenty to thirty people. The ship would moor close to various beaches that we were to clean, and we would go ashore during the day and return to the ship at night. During the first week or so, we had to go down into the bowels of the ship every morning where the landing boats were floating. When they started the diesel engines on all the landing craft, the air would be full of diesel exhaust from all those two-cycle engines. The procedure was to sink the stern of the ship until the landing craft could float out. Fortunately, after that first week or so, we started using a barge to get to the beaches.

During the first week, we spent most of our time sopping up oil with pompoms, but that wasn't very efficient. Then we got pumps that we carried to the beaches on our landing craft, along with other equipment we needed. When we hit a beach, we would string out the hose and pump water to the top of the beach to try to wash the oil down into the bay, where it would be collected by booms. Skimming boats would then pick up that oil. We used both hot and cold water on the beaches. Sometimes we even used steam generators to make steam for steam wands in an attempt to melt the oil off the rocks.

We wore gloves and tied our rain pants and jackets shut over our boots and wrists. Sometimes we wore plastic face shields, but it wasn't always practical to do that. If it was a cold day when we were using the steam wands to try to steam the oil off some of the rocky cliffs, our face shields would fog up. When that happened, we would just have to take them off so that we wouldn't risk falling off a cliff because we couldn't see. And, of course, without those face shields, we had to breathe even more of the oily fumes and our faces got splattered with oil.

We fell down quite a lot when we were working. At Green Island, the beach was covered with a mousse-like substance made up of oil and rotting seaweed. That was especially slippery, so you had to walk really carefully.

One of the things some of us tried at Green Island was to use high-pressure hoses to boil up the sand and gravel down deep to get out the oil that had sunk into the sand. We were getting out a lot more oil that way, so the skimmers had to come to our end of the beach more often. When the foreman realized what we were doing, he told us not to do that anymore because they just wanted to get the surface oil.

As soon as we started working on the spill cleanup, we all came down with a cough. We were given cough medicine, but it didn't help. We coughed all summer long because of the oil vapors. We could feel the congestion in our lungs. At other times in the past, I had worked around asphalt, applying heated grease and slapping on heavy grease, but that had never bothered me or made me cough the way this oil spill did.

During the first couple of months while I was working on the oil spell, I would get brown blisters on my lower legs that would pop and ooze a brown liquid, but those blisters disappeared by November. I was luckier than most people who worked on the oil spill because the exposures don't seem to have affected my health in a lasting way like they did the health of my two brothers.

*   *   *   *   *

Mike Potter

The union had negotiated our wages; we usually get extra around hazardous materials, but we didn't in this case. At least we got a lot of hours—seventeen-hour days a few times.

We felt nauseated all the time we were working out there on the beaches, and headaches were rampant. I think Exxon knew more about what warm weather spills did to people than what cold ones did. Then in addition to all the oil we were exposed to, there were a bunch of chemicals that we used. We would request and request that we be given the hazardous chemical plat that was supposed to be on top of the containers of chemicals, but we never could find out what ingredients were in the containers. We didn't have anything other than a name on the container. We nicknamed one of the chemicals we used Agent Orange. One of the things it was used for was to wash the oil off the boats and skiffs. That chemical was eating the membranes in people's noses. On our second or third R&R, word was getting out that if you were asked to work around this chemical, you should refuse to do it. That's why we wanted to get information about the chemicals we were using. Exxon knew a lot more than they wanted to tell us.

I started having some fairly serious memory loss problems a few years after the spill, even though I was only in my thirties. People would say, "Mike, how are you doing?" and I wouldn't recognize them. I used to know the phone numbers of people I call a lot. Now I have to look them up.

I developed some growths that looked like a huge wart. They were 3/4" thick and about the size of a silver dollar. Those big wart-like growths appeared about three years after I had worked on the oil-spill cleanup. A lot of my ailments started around 1993, about four years after the spill. That was when I started having some black-out spells and getting serious fatigue. We had signed an agreement that Exxon had the right to check our medical signs for thirty years. Doctors took blood and also did a urinalysis from time to time, but they never referred me to other doctors for any of my problems.

I was able to keep working fairly steadily until 2001, but then I had to shift to lighter work than construction because of my fatigue. I worked mainly as a mechanic, and some of the cleaning solvents I had to use made my arthritis a little worse. When I'm around chemicals, I have a lot more pain. I had to take early retirement at age forty-eight and get Social Security Disability Insurance.

* * * * *

Paul Potter, Deceased

Mike: I was on the same beach as my brother Paul where we were picking up debris like dead, oil-soaked wildlife that gave off a terrible rotten stench. We put this stuff in plastic bags to be picked up by a little barge, and these bags were sitting on the beaches in the hot sun. Usually the tops were twisted, but when Paul picked up this one bag, the top swirled open and gases poured out onto his face. He staggered around and said he couldn't see, so some guys had to grab him. They sent him to Anchorage on a helicopter, and he spent several days in a hospital there. The exposure kind of paralyzed his breathing. He got some of the stuff in one of his eyes and almost lost it; he was actually blind for a while. From that time on he always had white stuff in his tear duct. After that incident, almost any chemical would make Paul feel nauseated.

Teri, Paul's widow: After Paul finished working on the oil spill cleanup, he went back to doing carpentry work and building houses, but products he had used forever started bothering him. He even had a violent reaction to the gout medicine that he had taken off and on for many years. There were at least four times that he had to get medical attention because of exposure to something toxic. One time when he was putting a sealant on a deck, he got really sick and dizzy, so they had to take him to a clinic. They called a poison hot line and hooked him up to IVs to get him stabilized. Sometimes he would have a milder reaction, but he would still end up stuck in bed for a couple of days with a violent headache, feeling yucky and kind of weak. He would react to almost anything that was petroleum-based. Once when we were painting an apartment and using an oil-based primer on the walls, he almost passed out into the tray of paint. He had never reacted to things like that before the *Exxon Valdez* cleanup. He had built things off and on all his life.

Paul also had trouble with lung infections after he worked on the oil spill. He blamed his ill health on the spill cleanup work he had done.

At the time Paul died, the two of us were working as caretakers for an apartment complex. The week before he died he told me that the gas fumes from the snow blower were starting to make him sick. After that, I tried to get him to let me do all the snow blowing around the apartments. It was the man-thing though—he wouldn't let me do it. It was only a half hour after he came in from snow blowing one day that he had a massive heart attack. He died in the ambulance on the way to the hospital. His doctor said that the snow blower gas fumes were most likely what had killed him. Paul was only forty-four when he died.

Linda Baker

Coach and Physical Education Teacher

Pesticide poisoning was about the last thing on my mind on April 28, 1997, when I went as usual to the school where I taught. Eager to begin my day, I opened the door to the physical education office as I had done every Monday morning for sixteen years. What happened next changed the course of my life. A strong chemical smell that I later learned was pesticide hit me, immediately making me nauseous. Within a couple of minutes my hands became numb, my heart started beating erratically, and a migraine headache sickened me. It was hard to think logically, dizziness set in, and breathing became very difficult. On legs that felt too weak to hold me up, I stumbled up to the principal's office. Both secretaries got up to help me and asked what in the world that awful smell on my clothes was. It smelled like a cross between petroleum and ether to me, but I had no idea what it was. I had an overwhelming chemical taste in my mouth that no amount of mouthwash or toothpaste could get rid of for several days, but that was the least of my concerns.

It is no exaggeration to say that I felt like I was dying that day. I was unable to get my head clear and several times I thought it might be my last day on this earth because the chemicals triggered severe heart arrhythmias. I barely remember showering twice, trying to get rid of that chemical smell. I put the clothes I had removed in a garbage bag and set it in my laundry room to deal with later. My doctor told me emphatically that we had to find out exactly what I had been exposed to. The principal gave me the name of a pyrethrin insecticide that had been used; two and a half years later I found out that was not the full story. My doctor called a National Pesticide Hotline but learned of no specific treatment to help me, although he did advise me to stay away from further exposure to pesticide.

Being an active physical education teacher and coach, I assumed—incorrectly—that I might be sick the rest of the day but would be able to fulfill my teaching duties the rest of the week. Although I went back to work at noon the next day, I felt like I had a horrible flu all week. The day I went back to work, my mom called me at school to say, "Something terrible has happened at your house. When I opened the door, there was a very strong chemical smell." Just smelling the clothes I had left in the trash bag made her nauseous, so I told her to throw them away. Since I was still unable to enter the school building without severe symptoms returning, I taught outside the rest of the week. As it turned out, I taught outside through the end of that school year and into the first week of October of the following year, when I was forced to take a leave of absence.

To say I got no cooperation from the school administration is an understatement. These people had been my friends, so I was greatly disappointed to find that money meant much more to them than their employees. I was also appalled that they had so little concern for the students' health. If the pesticide could deck a healthy adult, what could it do to the children? They didn't seem to care. After much discussion, I finally talked them into hiring an industrial hygienist to check the building. They let him come but refused to let him bring any testing equipment. Thus I lost my only real chance to find out what pesticides I had been exposed to and at what levels.

Even though I repeatedly tried to re-enter the building and got sick time after time, the administrators kept trying to convince me—and everyone else—that my illness was "all in my head." I can still hear them saying, "You could go in that building if you thought you could." That hurt, as I had given them my best effort for sixteen years and had rarely taken a sick day. They also ignored a number of students who became ill with unusual symptoms: chest pains, head-to-toe rashes, severe stomach aches, migraine headaches, and difficulty concentrating. Some asthmatic kids had to bring their breathing machines to school.

The administration made it as tough on me as possible. I taught outdoors on 95-degree days, and they didn't even check to see if I had water. The area around a pine tree on the playground became my classroom. Other teachers and students brought out needed supplies, and my faithful friends would come out after school to check on me. But none of that was helping me get back into the building. I was forced to take a sick day every time it rained, and the business manager who supervised our self-funded health insurance refused to pay my medical bills. When I filed a workers' compensation claim, they fought it, even going so far as to bring in state school board attorneys.

It was my hope that the summer would bring healing and that I could start school as usual in the fall. I did regain some strength during the summer vacation, but that strength vanished when I returned because they had sprayed the school with pesticide the week before classes started. I gave it my best shot, but I just couldn't breathe inside that building. Pesticide exposure was wrecking my health and my career.

Not only was I forced to take a leave of absence, but I was also forced to see a workers' comp doctor who had a reputation of siding with employers. Fortunately, in my case he recognized the symptoms of pesticide poisoning and recommended that I be given a leave with pay until the projected new gym was built. This was my only hope of being able to teach again. By this point, I had learned that just prior to the day I had been poisoned, the business manager had ordered the entire building sprayed heavily and that pesticide residue had blanketed the building. If no pesticide was applied in the new gym, I was confident that I could return to teaching.

When the administration's own workers' comp doctor requested in writing that they use nontoxic building supplies and nontoxic pest control, I thought I had a chance. But the administration tried to discredit their own doctor by asserting that my physician brother had told him what to say. My brother did not, and would not, do anything like that, and I really resented their accusation that he had done something unethical. At this point, I was forced to see a second workers' comp doctor who had a fierce, business-friendly attitude. I was shocked when he walked in the room and said, "I don't work for you, the patient. I work for the insurance company." Even more shocking was the false report he wrote that included tests that I had never taken. But he made a big mistake. He said that I had had a normal chest x-ray. Since I had never had a chest x-ray, he was eventually caught in his lies. He was reported to the State Board of Healing Arts and received a reprimand.

As the months dragged on, the medical bills began to pile up, even though the string of doctors I saw really didn't know how to help me. I was now experiencing symptoms not only upon exposure to pesticide and herbicide, but also when I encountered a number of petroleum products, smoke, plastics, cleaning supplies, and virtually anything with a scent. At that point, I had never heard of multiple chemical sensitivity

(MCS). I didn't know what was happening to me, and neither did the doctors. The school district refused to pay my salary or my medical bills, so I went eight months without an income. It was quite humbling to have the other teachers take up a collection so that I would have money for food. Despite these difficulties, I continued to hold out the hope that I would be able to teach in the new building, and I had a series of meetings with district officials to make sure they knew how to keep the building safe for me.

When the first in-service day came in August of 1998, I was very excited to be going back to work. The administration had assured me that they had honored my requests for a nontoxic environment, so I thought that I was finally going to be able to teach again. I was disappointed beyond words when I entered the new gym that day and the pesticide-related symptoms began at once. They quickly became life-threatening, but I stayed in the gym as long as I could because I knew if I left this time, I was walking away from the career I loved.

Less than thirty minutes after I had entered the gym, I had to leave because my life was more important than my job. I stumbled onto the playground, thinking the fresh air would make me feel better. Even though I was barely able to comprehend what was going on around me, I was appalled to see that herbicide had been applied in wide circles under all the pieces of playground equipment. Herbicide had never been used on that playground in the sixteen years I had worked there, but they were making sure I couldn't even teach outdoors now. Nauseous, dizzy, breathing with great difficulty, and with my heart beating erratically, I made my way to a tree that I could lean against. A substitute teacher saw me and alerted the secretaries, who raced to my side. Afraid for my life, they put me in a van and rushed me to the doctor's office. I couldn't walk without help and felt like I was going to pass out at any moment. I spent the morning sprawled on an examining table, praying to live. I will never forget the look on the doctor's face when he came in. It is not a good thing to see fear on your doctor's face, but he could not hide his concern. I knew at that moment that pesticide had permanently ended my teaching career.

My doctor would not allow me to return to that toxic environment, but I was too sick anyway to even think about it. For the next eight months, I couldn't even walk across the room without help. For nearly a year, reading a newspaper was impossible because the words just didn't make sense to me. I remember trying to watch a football game and finally just turning toward the wall in tears because I couldn't figure out what was going on. This was a sport that I knew so well I had even been asked to coach it one year, and now I couldn't even watch a game. It took me over a year to build up enough strength to walk the 100 yards down the driveway to get my mail. My family and friends did my cooking and shopping and anything else that needed to be done around my house. This was all very distressing because I had formerly been a very active and independent individual. Before I got poisoned, I had twice gone on 5,000-mile solo camping trips. Now that was only a dream, and my goal each day was simply to survive. Many, many days I didn't know when I opened my eyes in the morning if I would live to see the sunset. My mom would come to my house and peek into the bedroom to see if I was still breathing. It was an extremely tough time for my whole family.

At last I heard about a doctor in Maryland who specializes in chemical injury cases. She is not only an M.D. but also has a doctorate degree from Harvard School of Public Health. I decided to go Maryland to seek her help because she knew how to treat pesticide poisoning. Although my teaching days were over, I was still fighting workers' comp and ADA claims, and I knew I would need this doctor's support in that effort.

As soon as I was strong enough to travel, I headed east. Since I was unable to stay in motels because of their use of pesticides and strong cleaning products, I packed my tent and camped my way back to Maryland. It was worth the trip to find a doctor devoted to helping those poisoned by pesticide and treating the chemical sensitivity that it so often triggers. She told me that I had all the signs of chlorpyrifos poisoning, even though the district was still maintaining that all they had used was a pyrethrin insecticide. (Pyrethrin is in fact a neurotoxic chemical that is capable of producing numbness, headaches, breathing difficulties, and allergic reactions. It is also a suspected sensitizer and endocrine-disruptor.) The physician also suspected I had been exposed to more than just a new finish on the gym floor on that day when I tried to return to school and got so sick. She immediately began trying to find out what I had really been exposed to. Her persistence paid off, and I was shocked at what she discovered.

Despite claims by district officials that no pesticide had ever been applied around the new gym, paperwork showed that nearly $2,000 worth of pesticide had been applied under the new addition, despite the fact that it was a concrete block building. We also have the paperwork to prove that not only had they used a pyrethrin insecticide the first day I was poisoned, but they had also used diazinon and chlorpyrifos. (Both of these last two pesticides have since been banned for indoor use because so many people have been poisoned by them.) A janitor who had no specific training in pest control and who by his own admission could barely read had applied the pesticides. Actually, his failure to keep the school clean had triggered the complaint that led to the business manager telling him to spray the building heavily. After he received this order, the janitor went to the school board office, grabbed three cans of pesticide left by pesticide salesmen, and applied them indiscriminately in the building. And he didn't just apply the pesticides to the baseboards. There was pesticide residue all over the pictures that had been hanging on my office wall. Clearly, these pesticides that would have been toxic even when applied using the best precautions had been mishandled and misapplied. We also learned that one of the pesticides he used had not been registered for sale in my state since 1989, but it was technically not illegal to apply it. Unethical, yes—illegal, no. It was particularly distressing to realize that children have very little protection from toxic pesticides applied in and around school buildings.

I called the State Agricultural Department to see if they had any jurisdiction over which pesticides were applied in schools. When they heard what had happened to me, they offered to come down and investigate the school building and interview people involved in the pesticide incident. Two investigators came to my home for what they thought would be a thirty-minute interview, and they left four hours later. They admitted that they had initially thought they were coming to "talk to another nut." But as they left, they both agreed that they had just talked to a true victim.

These officials went immediately to the school building and began to take samples and ask questions. This time the principal couldn't stop them. Although too much time had elapsed to get clear readings from the samples, they did discover one reason I had become so ill. My office had no back wall, but instead an open tunnel that ran under a hallway to the janitor's room. The janitor admitted he sometimes mixed up pesticide near a drain that led into the opening of that tunnel. He had either spilled or poured pesticide down that drain, and when the door to the janitor's room was opened, the positive pressure created had shoved the chemicals straight into my office. I had received a heavy dose of these pesticides, one that could easily have killed me.

Life over the next few years was extremely difficult. For nearly three years, I didn't leave my own house or yard because exposure to pesticide or herbicide made me deathly sick. My dad did all my grocery shopping, and friends often called to see if I needed anything when they went shopping out of town. I missed being able to attend church, and social events of any kind were out of the question. With my coaching background, I missed going to ball games, and that reality became nearly unbearable when I was forced to miss my nephews' high school basketball careers. Three years in a row I was too ill to spend Christmas with my family, and I also missed countless birthdays and other celebrations. I lived in isolation. I felt like I was in prison, even though I was not surrounded by bars. The barriers created by pesticide and herbicide were every bit as real.

Unfortunately, my mother also became chemically sensitive as a bizarre result of my pesticide poisoning event. Previously, she had never had an allergy of any type. Blessed with good health and limitless energy, she was an active person whom people half her age could not keep up with. All that changed the day she tried to clean the pesticide residue off the pictures from my office. She knew how much those pictures meant to me so she picked them up, spread them out on a sidewalk and began to scrub off the pesticide residue. She had to stop when she began to feel like she was coming down with the flu. She put the pictures in an old shed and took it easy for a few days until she felt better. In about a month, she once again spread the pictures out on a sunny sidewalk and began to clean them. As happened before, she soon felt like she had the flu. This time it was more severe and lasted longer. Severe nausea, stomach pains, and diarrhea sent her to the hospital, where they ran several tests. Of course, the tests were not designed to detect pesticide poisoning, and they all came up negative. It took her a long time to feel better, but she eventually did recover and tried to clean the pictures one more time because the connection between that pesticide residue and her illness was still not clear to her. But this time, she became so ill that there could be no doubt as to the cause of her illness. I told Mom to bury the pictures in a landfill, but it was too late to save her health. She also developed multiple chemical sensitivity as a result of exposure to the same pesticides that poisoned me. Like I had done, she camped her way back to Maryland to get help from the chemical injury doctor who had helped me so much.

My mom was not the only person besides me to be affected by the pesticide sprayed at school. A librarian and three aides had moved into my old office, and three of the four developed fibromyalgia and one developed breast cancer. Two of them had to have hysterectomies. A string of autoimmune diseases struck people in the building. Five were diagnosed with rheumatoid arthritis. One was told she had lupus, although her symptoms disappeared when she transferred to another building and was able to avoid pesticide exposures. Another teacher has peripheral neuropathy that threatens not only her job, but also her life. Diabetes, asthma, and allergies are common, as are migraine headaches. Three other people from the building are also on disability, and five have developed cancer. The special education teacher who taught just down the hall from me died of breast cancer. Depression, sleep disorders, pain syndromes, and breathing difficulties are common. Approximately 75 percent of the staff is dealing with some sort of chronic illness, even though the vast majority of people suffering with these illnesses would have rated their health as good or excellent prior to the pesticide application. I do not believe this is coincidental. Knowing the consequences of chemical exposures for adults, I shudder to think what it must be doing to all the children.

Although life was bleak for a long period after I first got so sick, the coach in me would not give up and the Christian part of me would not lose hope and faith. I thanked God every day that I had family, friends, and doctors who still believed in me and would do anything in their power to help me. Buoyed by their support, I gradually began to improve enough to start trying to educate others about the hazards of toxic pesticides and how to switch to nontoxic alternatives. A student teacher I had worked with the year before I got poisoned was now a principal and working toward his doctoral degree in education. He was aware of what happened to me and quite concerned about the people he was responsible for in his own building. He wanted to make sure he did everything in his power to protect them, so he decided to write his doctoral thesis on the problem of pesticides in schools and how schools could switch to nontoxic pest and weed control. I was honored when he asked me to help him with this project, and we spent many hours gathering information. We sent pesticide surveys to every school district in the state of Missouri and found that although some districts were committed to using only nontoxic pest control methods, many district superintendents and principals didn't even know what chemicals were being used or when they were applied.

Until more national protections are in place, my mother and I continue to work with local officials to reduce pesticide use in our community. After a five-year battle, the local school district switched to a nontoxic pesticide, but unfortunately, they have fallen back to their old ways of spraying toxic pesticides monthly. We continue to try to educate them about notoxic alternatives. Our city manager has instructed the Public Works Department to use only nontoxic pest and weed control. Our church also now uses only nontoxic pest and weed control, and they have also established a "fragrance-free" section that allows me and my mom to attend church again. The railroad gives us forty-eight-hour advance notice before they spray the tracks and leaves a three-block section of track near my mom's home unsprayed. The highway department also gives us forty-eight-hour advance notice of spraying near us and honors my request that no herbicide be used within a half mile of my home. My friends and family are very careful to be fragrance-free when they come to visit. They tease me about causing lots of "bad hair days."

I am especially grateful that a local state park where we have a little cabin made out of an old caboose is kept safe for us. The park manager has cooperated with us by switching to nontoxic pest and weed control, which allows us to use our cabin as a safe retreat during times of heavy herbicide use by homeowners in the city.

This little cabin has literally been a life-saver for me this year because I have not been able to live in my own home for the past ten months. Neighbors who had never sprayed anything toxic before this year recently decided to spray a fence row. That herbicide application kept me out of my home for about six weeks. I had only been back in my home for five nights before a new neighbor, who apparently did not understand the severity of my illness, used a very toxic pesticide to treat his property for termites. I became ill immediately. I keep my camping gear packed in my truck for just such emergencies, so I grabbed some food and water and left as quickly as possible. As I type this story, I am still not able to return home and do not know when that will be possible, if at all. I have lived in a tent a good portion of this year, but came to our cabin when it got too cold to live outdoors. I am so grateful to have a place to live that doesn't make me sick. Way too many people with multiple chemical sensitivity have nowhere to go to escape from chemical exposures.

I have always been a "people person," and the isolation forced upon me by MCS has been almost as difficult to deal with as the physical illness. I wondered how I would ever be able to interact with people and meet new friends when I was trapped in my own home. As I have been able to get out a little more, I have been amazed at how many people I have met are also struggling with pesticide poisoning and MCS. Make no mistake about this one point: anyone can be poisoned by a pesticide—anytime and anywhere.

So how has pesticide changed my life? It ruined my teaching career, my health, and my independence. It ruined my ability to enjoy simple pleasures like eating in a restaurant or attending sporting events. It has cost me well over $100,000 in medical bills and lost retirement benefits. I have missed out on family moments I will never get back. My normal life was turned upside down. The last thing on my mind that day in April when I was poisoned by the pesticide has now become the first thing on my mind because I must avoid pesticide exposure in all my daily activities. Before going anywhere, I must evaluate my chances of chemical exposures. If I guess wrong, I pay the consequences.

Fortunately, pesticide could not touch my faith or optimism or character or determination to make the best of my current situation. My life is now devoted to educating the public about the intolerable risk of pesticide exposures, and I pray daily that somehow I am making a difference. I know what a severe pesticide exposure did to me. I don't want it to happen to you.

Bonnie Giebfried

9/11 Emergency Medical Technician

In September of 2001, I was working as an EMT in the New York City 9-1-1 system. After the terrorist attack on the World Trade Center, we were one of the first units into the South Tower, and we got three people out of that building.

At this point, my partner Jen and I met up with a couple of our paramedics and their student, and this is when we started to see and hear the jumpers. When they hit the ground, it sounded like gunshots. We were told to move back, which we did, but we continued to witness the Twin Towers burning and the people jumping to their deaths. We were backing away from the falling debris when a loud noise rang out, the ground shook, and a ball of fire came at us. We ran up the grass and saw a little alcove on the side of the Financial Bulding that we thought was an entrance. Unfortunately, it wasn't. It was just a very small space where there had at one point been phone booths. We were trapped there when the gigantic fireball rolled by, pushing cars, trees, concrete, and everything else in its path.

The fireball buried thirty of us alive in that small space–emergency medical technicians, firefighters, police, and others. There were burning materials and debris around us. We tried so desperately to get out the way we came in, but the pile of debris blocking the entrance was worse than concrete. You couldn't even budge it. We started trying to break the windows that separated the alcove from the Financial Building, but the windows were heavily reinforced with several thick panes of glass. The air was getting very thin in this small space because everything was burning, superheated. I could hear my heart beating, and people were stopping breathing. At that point, I said, "God, take care of my friends and my family" and closed my eyes, expecting to die. Then I heard pop, pop, pop because Lieutenant McGinn, one of the police officers trapped with us, succeeded in shooting out the windows separating us from the Financial Building. Suddenly there was air to breathe, and we could get into the building.

After we got into the Financial Building, everyone started to scatter, trying to find a way out to the street. It was dark beyond belief; you could hardly see. After our experience of having been virtually buried by the wall of debris, we all threw up this stuff that we had swallowed. God knows what it was–bits of trees, furniture, concrete–anything that had been swept up by the fireball that rolled past us.

When we finally got out of the Financial Building, we went into a nearby deli. We had no idea the South Tower had collapsed and was gone; we just thought the top had blown off from the explosion. Everyone's eyes were burning from the smoke, dust, and debris. People started to come into the deli, and we went into EMT mode again and started to triage breathing problems and injuries like broken arms, abrasions, and contusions. After a while, my partner Jen and I made the decision to leave the deli because we thought the building might be unstable.

We went to a medical van nearby to get more supplies and then started walking down the street. All of a sudden the ground started shaking again, just as it had when the South Tower collapsed. We dropped everything and ran into an underground parking garage. The debris started coming at us, and once again it blocked the entrance we had just gone in.

After the debris had settled a bit, Jen pulled her flashlight out because we couldn't see three feet in front of us. Then we heard people calling, "Is anyone in here?" We called to them to move toward our voices and look for the light. We met up with a police officer and four other people, and we all kicked our way through the debris that was blocking the entrance to the parking garage. The police officer told us to go toward the water, so we headed there.

When we reached the water, Jen and I set up a makeshift triage area and started treating anyone who came to us for assistance. More resources were arriving, and a fireboat pulled against the sea wall where we were. We directed the emergency cases to the fireboat. By this point, all kinds of other boats were also coming to assist in getting people off the island. In the midst of all that was going on, I began to feel ill and my breathing got really bad. I sat down because I was getting very weak, and Jen ran to find albuteral because I was having a severe asthma attack.

I had never had asthma before 9/11, but by the end of the day I had had three bad asthma attacks. That feeling of not being able to catch your breath, not being able to fill your lungs, is such a horrible, horrible feeling. It feels like someone's crushing your chest, sucking everything out of you.

Before long we were redeployed to the North Cove Marina, but shortly after we arrived at the marina, we were told there was a threat of a gas explosion. At this point we made a decision to get on the boat to evacuate to New Jersey.

The albuteral treatment had not broken my asthma attack, and I was starting to have another attack as the boat sped away from the marina. When I told Jen that I was having another asthma attack, she said, "There's no oxygen on the boat; just keep breathing!" All I could see as we crossed the river was the city burning under a thick black cloud of smoke to the left of me and the Statue of Liberty to the right of me.

By the time we reached New Jersey, I could hardly stand up. Two men grabbed under my arms and brought me up the walkway, where an ambulance crew took me to their unit to be treated. The paramedics gave me another treatment of albuteral, but it wasn't breaking the attack, so they had to start an IV and give me a steroid (salmuetral) to help stop the chest pain and asthma attack I was having.

The World Trade Center attack changed my life forever in profound ways. Before 9/11, I was in great health. I was playing on three soccer teams, three softball teams, a racquet ball league, a paddle ball league. I was fishing, hiking, climbing mountains. Just before 9/11 I had climbed my first 13,000-foot peak in Colorado, and I was aspiring to climb the 14,000-foot peaks in Colorado. I can't even climb up stairs now. I just can't catch my breath. I have chronic sinusitis, bronchitis, asthma. I just got over having pneumonia for the third time. Never had pneumonia before 9/11. Now my doctors are concerned about my heart because severe asthma attacks and the requisite medications can produce heart problems.

I was thirty-seven when the terrorist attack on the World Trade Center occurred and was looking forward to a full and productive life. Now I'm forty-four years old, but I feel like a ninety-year-old. My muscles are atrophying. Anytime that the media is around they ask, "Well, how can you attribute this to 9/11?" Sorry, my friend and co-worker Tim Keller was less than a foot from me. Tim Keller is dead.

Paramedics Felix Hernandez and Debbie Reeve, who were working with us that day, are dead. They weren't old individuals. They were in their thirties when they responded on 9/11, but all three were dead five years later from causes their paramedics' union related to the toxic exposures at Ground Zero.

The chronic health problems I have developed because of everything I breathed in on 9/11 have made it impossible for me to continue my work as an emergency medical technician. That has been a big loss in my life because it was a profession I loved. I'm also struggling financially now. I was making sixty grand before 9/11. Now I'm over sixty grand in the hole.

Since 9/11, I've become very sensitive to various chemicals that never used to bother me, so I have to be really careful what I expose myself to. The other night I went out for Japanese food, which is one of my favorite things to do. I was having a good time with my life partner when this guy came in who was wearing a lot of cologne. My throat started closing up, and I began to get chest pains. I had to leave the restaurant, which was really disappointing. On other occasions, perfume exposure in a restaurant has caused me to become nauseated. People don't realize that there's more involved with the health problems we developed at Ground Zero than just the physical injury, the respiratory injury, the psychological problems. The multiple chemical sensitivity issues that have come from 9/11 have not been addressed.

I can't do normal, everyday things because of my chemical sensitivity. I really have to police myself to make sure that I'm not going to be exposed to gas fumes or the propane for the barbeque. Household cleaners–Oh, my God, you just might as well pack me up at that point and send me to the hospital.

It's torture. You know, some days you wish you'd died that day because living–I don't call this living. Part of me died 9/11. I will never get that back, and since that terrible terrorist attack, I've been just existing day in, day out.

Daniel Brainerd

Student

My son Daniel committed suicide in 2005. What makes his life note-worthy is the way he had to live it. In the fall of 1993, Daniel was a nine-year-old student in the fourth grade at Blakely Elementary School on Bainbridge Island, Washington. His life was irrevocably changed that fall by his exposure to chemicals used in the renovation at his school. Prior to this time, Daniel had been so healthy that he had never been to the doctor except for check-ups and immunizations.

During the summer of 1993, the grade school underwent a massive renovation. To keep the asbestos in the old linoleum tiles from becoming airborne, solvents were used to remove the floor tiles. These solvents were absorbed into the concrete below and into the surrounding wallboards. Petroleum naphtha was one of the primary substances in the solvent. The renovation was finished just a few days before school started; new laminate, carpeting, and paint in a building that was built in the 1970s made for a very toxic environment. The smell of chemicals struck anyone who stepped inside. When I volunteered in my son's classroom that fall, I felt some effects but thought I just had a cold or other illness.

Although more than a dozen students and teachers reported adverse symptoms related to the chemical exposure, these reports were labeled "group hysteria." School officials were quick to claim that the situation was not "unhealthy" and did everything possible to prove it. It took over eighteen months before school officials acknowledged the situation and took even limited action. A year after the renovation, one teacher had cancerous nodes removed from his vocal cords; another was diagnosed with lupus, and another with asthma.

In the first few days of the exposure to chemicals in his school environment, my son Daniel suffered severe stomach pain. He would lie curled up in bed, crying. After a few weeks at school, his lymph nodes were swollen to the size of pecans, and his skin was pale. There was no color on his ears, which now looked as if they were made of wax. Blood tests showed nothing. Daniel's doctor conferred with a colleague in the Department of Environmental Science at the University of Washington. At his suggestion, our doctor wrote a letter to the school, recommending that my son be placed near an open window to help alleviate his symptoms.

Daniel experienced so much fatigue that he would sleep up to eighteen hours a day. I often had to wake him to eat dinner. In the past, he had eaten enough to choke a horse; now he ate barely anything and complained that food tasted funny. Red meat tasted metallic to him, and he just wasn't hungry. He had been a slim boy, weighing sixty-nine pounds, but because of his loss of appetite, he lost seven pounds in five months. By spring he looked like an AIDS patient. His ribcage was visible, and he had so little energy that he couldn't ride his bike for more than five minutes at a time. His physical symptoms were alarming enough, but some of changes in his personality were even harder to bear. My once lively, super-charged, completely upbeat child was reduced to a quiet, lethargic lump on the coach. His class was instructed to keep a journal, and it captured what he was experiencing as his former good health slipped away:

September 27: "I've been feeling very weird. I think I'm going to die for some reason."

September 28: "Today I've been sick to my stomach. Very low and bored."

October 3: " I haven't been doing well in school, I think its because I've been really tired."

After several months, Daniel began to have nosebleeds more and more often, and sometimes they lasted through the night. He got no relief from analgesics for his headaches, and antacids did nothing for his stomach. His symptoms would get better over the weekend, but after a week back in school, his symptoms would be worse than ever. I had no idea, however, that the health effects from the renovation would last his lifetime. I ignorantly thought, as did everyone around me, "It will pass; he'll get better." But weeks turned into months, and then the years passed and Daniel did not recover.

A few months after Daniel's initial exposure in his school, his symptoms started occurring in response to common chemical exposures in everyday situations. Over the course of two years, the extent of his disease became very apparent. Our only recourse was to avoid places that did not have good air quality–stores, certain houses, cars, etc. Daniel experienced the fewest symptoms when he stayed in his room with an air cleaner running. He did a lot of reading, and I finally gave into the computer game craze. It was one of the few things he could still do. He had lost the energy to take part in sports and dance.

In the months that followed Daniel's exposure and subsequent illness, I tried to work with his school to address the problem. The district hired experts to measure the levels of chemicals in the classrooms, and they tried to bake out the fumes during the weekends. The overall message was that the school was "safe." Parents' concerns continued to be attributed to mass hysteria. The hardest part of going through this experience was the lack of understanding even from friends and family members. The idea that our environment can sometimes be unsafe was more than most people were willing to accept. I was very alone as I fought my battle, sustained only by the knowledge that I was right. I knew my son was not psychosomatic, and I knew he was becoming more and more ill. On top of the illness from the chemicals, his immune system could no longer fight colds and flu. Always in the past, he would go to bed early when he felt a little sick and wake up the next morning completely over it. That first year after the renovation, he had the flu three times, and each time it took longer and longer to recover.

Feeling mounting frustration with the school officials, I turned my attention to things I could control. I educated myself and read all about green living. I took great efforts to make our houses as free as possible from volatile organic compounds (VOCs). I installed industry-quality water filters and air filters, used non-VOC paints and finishes, and learned to lay tile so I wouldn't have to use vinyl flooring or carpeting. I bought carbon-filter air cleaners.

Daniel resorted to wearing a cannister gas mask to reduce his symptoms in the car and outside when he was near cars. His nosebleeds stopped almost completely as a result, and he no longer had stomach aches after riding in the car. But he endured years of harassment about wearing the mask, not only from kids but from police as well. Security at a concert forced him to throw his mask away before they would allow him in. After that exposure at the concert, he was bedridden for four days, unable to eat and in severe pain. Sometimes he chose to endure a reaction from exposure rather than face the ridicule of the public. Daniel was even targeted as a threat because he was seen mailing a letter with his gas mask on; police came to the house to investigate him.

Ever since he became sick when he was in the fourth grade, Daniel was not able to attend school for more than two hours a day. He was classified as a health-impaired student, which entitled him to certain special education services. The school district that we lived in refused to accommodate him, however, and I had to take legal action several times to ensure his education. Each time I prevailed, but it required many months and a substantial outlay of funds. When we moved to New Jersey, we tried having him attend school as a regular student, but after a week it was clear that his health was not strong enough. I ordered his school records from Washington but really didn't expect much accommodation from his new school. I was surprised when not only did they readily accept his classification, they provided qualified tutors and I didn't have to fight to get him help.

As you can imagine, Daniel did not lead a normal life. He was limited by his illness and was unable to do many ordinary things. It was not easy for him to take part in after-school activities or just hang out with friends at the movies because the exposures he encountered would put him over his threshold. His life became quite empty because it was so hard for him to socialize. Daniel had one close friend from early childhood and made a few friends when he joined the computer club at the high school. They would take turns hosting the meetings at people's homes, playing computer games and sharing programming ideas. Despite the limitations of his life, I hoped that Daniel would eventually regain enough of his health to lead a normal life.

When Daniel was fourteen years old, I happened to watch him pick up something in the kitchen, and my heart dropped to my stomach. He was shaking as he lifted the object. I had noticed how bad his handwriting was becoming but hadn't really thought much about it until then. When I sent him for neurological testing, the neurologist concluded that his tremors, which occurred all over his body, not just his hands, were what are termed nonspecific. In other words, the neurologist could relate Daniel's tremors to no disorder, but said my fourteen-year-old son was experiencing the same type of tremors that appear in geriatric patients.

Daniel and I used to talk about all the ways he could improve his health and strategies for dealing with his illness. I bought lots of vitamins, antioxidants, and organically grown food, despite the cost. He dutifully took the vitamins, and unlike most teenagers, he ate a very good diet. He would save up his "exposure" time so he could go to a friend's house for a while. He was very cooperative with most of the changes that were necessary in his life, but it was clear that his deepest desire was just to be normal, to be able to go places and do things like all his friends.

Shopping was such a hassle because of the formaldehyde and other chemicals in the various products. Daniel would run into a store after I had checked it out and told him where to find the things he wanted to buy. He would quickly pick some things out and run back outside. Sometimes I would buy a bunch of things and bring them home for him to choose which he wanted. I watched him slowly withdrawing from activities outside of our home because it was just easier to stay home and avoid getting sick. The cost of a bad exposure was not just feeling lousy for the few minutes that he was exposed; it was days of torturous pain that few people acknowledged existed.

When Daniel finally went to college, he took some of his courses through correspondence to reduce the time he would need to be on campus. After Daniel moved out to room with a friend, there were two things I especially worried about. One was that he would live a lifestyle typical of other young men, which would be risky, given his chemical sensitivity. The other was that Daniel would be unable to self-monitor his emotional well-being. In fact, he was still very self aware, and even up to the time he committed suicide, he was still going running and getting his laundry done. I often e-mailed him notes to encourage him and say that if he needed anything he should let me know.

In 2004, eleven years after Daniel's health was so severely impacted by the renovation in his school, his liability lawsuit was finally settled out of court with the four defendants—the abatement company, the chemical company, the school district, and the managing contractor. The monetary cost and time invested in all the litigation had been very extensive.

The settlement gave Daniel some money, but it could not give him back his life. On November 29, 2005, he decided he could no longer deal with living in such a restricted way. The helplessness of his situation, the isolation he felt, and the sheer weight of dealing with such a limiting illness led to his suicide. As a young boy of five, he once told me he knew he wanted to be a dad of five children and then with some thought, he added: "Well, maybe just two for starters!" It's still hard for me to accept that even after a painful twelve-year struggle, he had decided that there was no way he could make life work for him.

Editor's Note: This story was written by Daniel's mother, Sara Cramer.

Bobbie Lively-Diebold

EPA Scientist

In 1985, I left my job at the United States Environmental Protection Agency in Region V, Chicago, and went to Washington, D.C., with my husband, a physicist who had just been hired by the Department of Energy. I found a new job in the Superfund program at the EPA headquarters, which was located in the Waterside Mall. This building had been constructed to be a shopping mall, not an office building, and the EPA leased it from a private company. There were still retail shops and restaurants on the first level, with the EPA offices on the upper floors and in an adjacent tower. The converted mall had many deficiencies. One major problem was that there were few windows in the building and those few did not open. In addition, the ventilation system did not operate properly because of its low air intake and poor air circulation.

After I had worked there for two years, the EPA began renovating an area of the building near where I worked. Walls were painted, new carpet was installed, and spaces were reconfigured with new furniture and space dividers for an open plan. Employees working in areas to be remodeled were moved to other areas, but many people had to keep working in areas close to where the renovation was taking place. The fumes from the various remodeling projects spread to these adjacent areas, and the ventilation system circulated them throughout the rest of the building.

Early in the morning on January 22, 1988, soon after the renovation had begun and the new carpet had been installed, I entered my office and smelled a strong, acrid chemical smell. Almost immediately, I began coughing and felt dizzy and nauseated. My breathing became labored, and my lungs started to hurt. In addition, I was disoriented and lost my voice. I left the office and remained outside until my head was clear enough that I could drive home.

After staying out of work for a few days, I felt somewhat better, and my supervisor, who was very supportive, arranged for me to work in various spaces in the Waterside Mall building that had not been remodeled. After a few hours in each of these spaces, however, I became ill and nauseated, could only speak in a very hoarse voice, and experienced mental confusion and lung pain. This was hardly surprising because the HVAC system was of course circulating air from the renovated portions of the mall to the non-renovated portions.

It was soon clear that I could not work in any space provided for me in the Waterside Mall. I was somewhat better at home on weekends, however. An occupational health physician documented my condition as being work related, and I applied for workers' compensation and received six weeks off through that program. After I spent six weeks at home, primarily in bed, some of my symptoms became less intense and my voice returned.

As the renovation continued and more new carpet was installed, more employees became ill. A number of affected employees got in touch with each other to compare symptoms and working conditions and formed an organization called the Committee of Poisoned Employees (COPE) that held weekly meetings. COPE members had a wide variety of professions and skills; the group included lawyers, toxicologists, analysts, public participation specialists, and regulators. EPA representatives of federal unions worked with COPE to inform other employees about the sick building problems at the Waterside Mall, various health symptoms that could be related to the renovation, and some steps that employees could take to avoid developing health problems. The union representatives also met with EPA building managers to obtain some relief, such as increasing air intake in the ventilation systems and providing safe work spaces for employees who had developed serious health problems.

Air quality tests by the EPA's emergency response team found that the new carpet was out gassing a chemical called 4-phenylcyclohexane (4-PC). These fumes released by the carpet were a likely cause of various neurological problems, lung pain, confusion, nausea, and loss of memory among employees. In later tests of carpet fumes on rats that were performed by Dr. Rosalind Anderson of Anderson Laboratories, the rats exhibited problems similar to those of the EPA employees. Some rats in the test even died from exposure to the fumes from carpets.

While I was out on workers' compensation, my program had been moved to another space in the Waterside Mall while our old space was being renovated. My occupational health doctor had advised my supervisor and other EPA officials that I could only work in a space where the air exchange was high enough to protect my health. Unfortunately, there wasn't any place in the building where this amount of air flow could be provided. To keep my job, I had no choice but to return to work with my section. But as the days passed, I had increasing problems. It was clear that I was not going to be able to work in that atmosphere very long.

I returned from lunch one day to find that carpet was being installed in an area several hundred feet away from our section. Shortly after I entered the building, I had an even stronger attack than the one I had experienced in January. I gasped for breath, my lungs burned, my face turned bright red, my heart beat irregularly, I was confused and disoriented, and I couldn't talk. Someone helped me to an elevator, and I stumbled outside the building. Unable to walk, I sat down on the ground next to a pillar in the rain. Some of the people who walked by asked me if something was wrong and if they could help me. I stayed in the rain for a long time too dazed to do or say anything. Somehow I managed to get home, and that was the last time I entered the Waterside Mall.

My occupational health doctor sent me to consult with some other doctors about some of my symptoms. I was told to avoid chemical exposures as much as possible; this seemed to be the only treatment available for my condition. Perfume and scented products made me violently ill. I could not pump gas for my car or do many of the tasks of everyday life that most people take for granted. Walking down the grocery aisle where soaps and cleaning products were displayed made me quite ill. My husband had to do most of the grocery shopping and all the vacuuming and cleaning at home. At this point, I was so fatigued that I stayed in bed except to go to the bathroom and to medical appointments. When I was in a car, I had to wear a respirator containing charcoal cartridges to protect myself from the traffic exhaust. I sometimes had episodes at a doctor's office where exposures in that atmosphere would cause one of my arms to start shaking violently or I would become nauseated or feel very ill. Somewhere along the line, the folks in our COPE group did some research and found that there was a name for our condition–multiple chemical sensitivity (MCS).

I used all my sick leave and annual leave and then applied again for workers' compensation and received it once again. After a year of being away from the Waterside Mall building, my health began to improve. Nevertheless, I was starting to have heart arrhythmias and would be sick for days or weeks whenever I was exposed to any type of volatile organic compounds (VOCs). Because of these reactions, I was quite isolated and usually saw only my husband, doctors, or other members of COPE. Occasionally, however, I would speak at an outdoor rally sponsored by the federal unions to bring pressure on EPA managers to provide better work conditions for all its employees, both well and sick.

Before long the press began to focus on how ironic it was that several hundred employees had become ill because of remodeling at the EPA, the very agency that was supposed to protect human health and the environment. Since I had no job to protect and there wasn't much else that the EPA could do to me, I agreed to be interviewed by the *Washington Post* and the *Washington Times*. I also made television appearances on "Good Morning America," "Larry King Live," the "Today Show," and "60 Minutes." Most of these programs were shot inside or just outside my home because I couldn't tolerate the exposures in TV studios. My goal in doing these interviews was to create awareness of the health problems, including MCS, caused by poor indoor air quality in sick buildings.

Meanwhile, the sick building problem continued at the EPA. The number of employees with health problems rose to at least three or four hundred. Once an employee became sick in an area, the EPA would move them out and move in a new employee without telling the new person about the reactions that some previous employees had experienced in this work setting. The new employees often developed chemical sensitivity in this situation, and the cycle continued.

For the first year after I left EPA, I lived at home in the one room that I could tolerate, which we closed off from the rest of the house. I used several air filters to clean the air, and we hired industrial hygienists to pinpoint chemicals and off-gassing in our house and make recommendations for improving our air quality. Eventually I was able to live in the whole house and sleep in our bedroom once again.

During my second year away from work, I kept urging the EPA management to allow me to work at home. I met the criteria for being handicapped and filed papers to be declared so. This allowed me to apply for reasonable accommodation under the Americans with Disabilities Act of 1990. I was told, however, that I could not work in my old job or any other job in Superfund since I would have to be in the building to do so. My résumé was circulated in the EPA's Office of Emergency and Remedial Response, and because of my prior excellent work history, I was offered a job in the Oil Program, developing and revising regulations for oil spill protection.

I returned to work in the beginning of 1990. EPA had set up a supposedly "clean" office space in another building where affected employees could work. Unfortunately, after an hour or two in that space, I had reactions and could not work there, although some chemically sensitive employees were able to do so. My only chance to work safely was to work at home, so the EPA finally provided equipment for me to work from my home with phones, a computer, and contractor support.

My job was to oversee the development of regulations to implement "The Oil Pollution Act of 1990." Once a week I met with my supervisor in a park outside EPA, and I kept in touch at other times by phone and computer. To minimize out-gassing, my branch chief provided me with a used computer and a printer with a typewriter ribbon, but I still had reactions to the computer. When I used it, my face would turn bright red and would burn and swell. For a number of months, I could avoid these reactions only by using a respirator when I worked on the computer. Even under these circumstances, I was able to accomplish a lot, and I participated in my supervisors' weekly branch meetings by conference phone. I was thus able to keep up with other projects going on in my office as well as to share information about my work. My supervisors were pleased with my work, and the arrangement seemed to function to everyone's advantage.

*   *   *   *   *

In 1992 our COPE group and the unions were approached by a law firm to discuss the possibility of the chemically injured employees suing the building management since those of us who had received workers' compensation could not sue the EPA. The affected employees agreed to enter the suit with the law firm on a contingency basis. Based on a review of our health records, the law firm chose five of the most highly affected employees and one spouse to initiate the lawsuit against the owner of the Waterside Mall. Among other charges, the lawsuit stated that the Waterside Mall lacked sufficient ventilation to conform to minimum industry standards and that the building owner's supervision of renovations at EPA Headquarters did not satisfy the applicable standard of care.

To get intensive medical examinations to document the extent of our injuries, the law firm sent us to a toxicologist, who tested us for many things, including oxygen flow to the brain, balance and inner ear problems, neurological damage, heart damage, and diminished concentration. My diagnosis from these and other tests was that I had toxic encephalopathy (a condition that occurs when there has been an alteration to the brain and central nervous system function as the result of exposure to various toxins). The tests also showed decreased oxygen flow to the thalamic area of my brain and provided evidence of both central and peripheral nervous system dysfunction.

Despite these tests, during our trial in the Superior Court of the District of Columbia, the jury refused to believe that four of the five of us were actually sick and considered our cases to be somatization. Nevertheless, they gave low monetary awards to all five of us EPA employees and the one spouse. The judge then tried to take away these monetary awards, but his decision was eventually overturned and our case was settled in 2001 on a confidential basis, almost a decade after it had begun.

While this legal battle was proceeding, I had to travel to various EPA regional offices in 1996 and 1997 to conduct Oil Facility Inspection Training that I was in charge of developing. I was usually gone for a week at a time. Although I was very careful about using an air filter in hotel rooms and in the training areas, as time went on I became sicker and extremely fatigued. I often had to work from my bed. My speech and movement problems occurred more frequently, as did shortness of breath and extreme fatigue. My chest inflamation continued, and nothing would reduce the pain. Walking up a flight of stairs left me breathless and unable to talk. I realized that my mental sharpness was slipping and I was having difficulty concentrating. I finally decided that I could not work any longer, and I retired in February of 1998. My supervisors and program were sad to see me go and told me that I managed to get more work done with fewer resources than anyone else.

Once I retired I had time to get medical help. I was referred to an electro-cardiologist who was familiar with chronic fatigue syndrome and had worked with patients with MCS. After various tests, the cardiologist found that I had damage to my small-vessel vascular system that caused the vessels to leak fluid into the surrounding tissue. When I was exposed to chemicals or other triggers, my body would become inflamed. The inflammation caused my veins to contract and my red blood cells to stick together, which made my heart work overtime. When parts of my brain did not receive enough oxygen, my speech would slur and the left side of my body would shut down. My heart had enlarged from all the extra strain, and I had a left branch bundle block. My blood vessels would fluctuate widely from being dilated to constricted, and this would cause headaches and circulatory problems.

After my health was stabilized to some degree, my husband and I began hunting for a house located in the country. I needed better outdoor air quality and enough acreage so I would be more protected from my neighbors' perfumed fabric softeners and wood smoke, as well as from auto exhaust. We searched for houses for a year but could not find a house that I was able to tolerate without becoming ill. Finally, we decided to build a "healthy house" that I could tolerate. We looked for months before we found a forty-seven-acre parcel in the Shenandoah Valley that we liked.

We hired an architect to design us a healthy house that used very few materials containing volatile organic compounds and included a state-of-the-art ventilation system. Our air exchange system recovers heat and cool air and recirculates all the air in the house to the outside every three hours. When we moved into the house in February of 2003, I did not have any problems from the new construction. If a neighbor is burning something outside, however, we turn off the air exchange system to avoid getting smoke into the house. During the four years we have lived in the house, my health has stabilized, although I still have severe reactions when subjected to an exposure while shopping or traveling. Once when a neighbor had his fields sprayed with herbicides, both the left and the right sides of my body shut down and I couldn't talk normally for five days. I could not walk and had the too familiar pain, confusion, and other symptoms from this herbicide exposure.

I limit my trips from the house and stay inside when the air quality is bad. I am not always able to attend family functions such as weddings because of renovations in hotels and churches. Through all these problems, however, my husband has stood by my side and supported me both literally and figuratively. He helps with the work when I am unable to do it, and he has welcomed EPA friends who have come to our houses for meetings and dinners and sometimes to live with us until their health has improved. In spite of my disability and MCS, I am fortunate that I can now function in a somewhat normal, albeit limited, degree, I have the love and support of my family, and I have been able to retire and live in a house that protects my health.

Sp4c. Tara Batista

Gulf War Veteran

I'm thirty-seven years old, and I have Gulf War syndrome. I joined the Army when I was eighteen right after I graduated from high school. I was trained to be a combat medic and to drive an ambulance.

Within a year or so after I enlisted, my unit was sent to the Persian Gulf. In preparation for our deployment, a civilian crew was hired to paint our vehicles with CARC (chemical agent resistant coating) paint, which is toxic and highly carcinogenic. One day our sergeant decided to have us to paint the numbers on our trucks using this paint. Now, the civilian painters wore protective suits and respirators, and they worked in big bays that vented the fumes out the top of the building. A group of us were in the motor pool building when the sergeant took the cover off a five-gallon can of CARC paint. I immediately reacted with pain behind my left eye, dizziness, and dry heaving. I also couldn't see well and fell to the ground. The sergeant said that just for that I had to paint all the numbers on the trucks. He left only one person to help me. I got a surgical mask out of my truck to give myself a little protection, but I was given no gloves to wear and no protective suit or respirator. By the time I was done with the last truck, I was covered with the CARC paint. It was days before it wore off. The other platoons went to the PX and bought ordinary spray paint to paint the numbers on the theory that the numbers didn't really have to be chemically resistant.

We deployed to Saudi Arabia right after Thanksgiving of 1990. After we arrived, we picked up our vehicles at the port. I drove a truck back to Cement City, where we were staying, and I developed a severe headache and vomited for hours, even while I was still driving back. When we reached Cement City, the guy in the truck with me had to half carry me to the tent. I had to take an antiemetic and two liters of fluid at the aid station.

After leaving Cement City, we went to a place called Log Base Victor. My battalion commander was there, along with a medical unit. On our first night there we were herded into a tent with guards at the door. They had ammo in their weapons, and I thought it was strange that some guards had weapons that were not in safety mode. The battalion commander jumped up on a table and said to us, "The shots you are about to get are top secret. Don't write home about it, don't tell people about this on the phone. There will be no record of you receiving it." They had us take our shirts off and get Vaccination A. Later I found out it was for anthrax. That night they also handed out pyridiostigmine bromide (PB) pills in a little white box to each of us and said we would get instructions on taking them at a later point.

There were numerous air raid sirens sounding, which meant that some kind of munition was traveling through the air. One of my jobs was to set up M8 alarms that detect nerve agent. These alarms kept going off, even though no one was near them and there were no vehicles whose exhaust could set them off. On one occasion when the alarms sounded, I put on MOPP 4, my chemical suit, and my gas mask and went to one corner of our site to sample the air with a 256 kit that detects if any nerve agent is in the area. The battalion commander was there and asked what I was doing. When I told him that my job was to check to see if there was a nerve agent in the area, he yelled at me to go back to my tent. An order is an order, so I had to leave.

One night we were told to line up outside the tent and to bring our PB pills and a canteen. The officers went from person to person. The sergeant had a tongue depressor, a red-lensed flashlight, and a bag, and the commander had a 9mm pistol in her hand. We got the idea and took the pills without asking any questions. They really affected our night vision because the drug causes constricted pupils. People also started behaving strangely.

One day we were attacked by five SCUD missiles. The Patriot missiles blew three of the SCUDs up, and the debris rained down on our area. Two others just hit somewhere in the desert. Not long after that SCUD attack, I started having strange symptoms. I felt very tired, my joints started aching, I became really forgetful, and I had episodes of incontinence. I didn't tell anyone about the incontinence; I was only twenty years old and it was just too embarrassing.

The war ended soon after this, and we headed south so that we could move into Khobar Towers in order to clean our equipment, which is difficult to do in a tent in the desert. Since our battalion commander was frequently in trouble with the 62nd med group, we ended up in some abandoned chicken coops. I happened to be within earshot when a captain who was apparently an environmental medical officer showed up and began speaking to the battalion commander. The captain explained that chicken waste can cause all sorts of respiratory and sinus issues and that it contains endospores that can cause illness. Other units had considered housing troops there, but had decided it just wasn't sanitary. The captain said that was why they were using the Khobar Towers as a place where units could clean their gear so they could clear customs. Unfortunately, the battalion commander basically told this captain that he outranked him and he would put his troops wherever he wanted. We stayed there.

When we opened the door of the first building, we saw a mountain of chicken droppings on a cement floor. There were big windows and a space between the cinder block walls and tin roof. They sent us to get pick axes, shovels, and wheelbarrows. When we started chipping that stuff off the floor, we realized pretty quickly that the dust we were creating was bad to breathe. It was absolutely disgusting. I tried putting a wet cloth over my nose and mouth, but it didn't help much at all.

Cleaning the chicken droppings off the cement floor was a huge problem because the stuff stuck like glue. Someone got the idea of spraying water under pressure on the floor, but that didn't work either. All we ended up with was chicken-dropping soup. Next the battalion commander filled some cement trucks with water and added a very strong bleach to the water, thinking that bleach will kill anything.

They hosed the bleach solution into the chicken coops, but it all came pouring right back out the door. Then they sent me to the motor pool to get sledge hammers. They had us knock holes in the walls every so many feet, thinking they could shoot the water in all the holes so it would spread out and clean the floor better. That didn't work either; the water just ran back out the holes.

Next they sent me and three other females to the motor pool to get some brooms and mops. They made us go into the chicken coop and scrub the floor while they pumped the water that contained bleach into the building. When I started scrubbing, I was soon enveloped in a white mist. I began having trouble breathing, and it felt like my trachea was being squeezed shut. I started having trouble seeing, and everything turned greenish yellow. When I started to cough up and vomit up frothy white stuff, I was afraid I was going to die. I fell out the door onto the sand, but the sergeant said, "Get the f___ back in there and finish." I refused to go back in. At that point, the officers in charge decided that whatever was left on the floors could stay there. They did not use the bleach solution in the other three chicken coops.

The area where we were located was an agricultural hub. There were a lot of cattle, goats, and chickens in the area, so there were water holes all over, which meant that the mosquitoes were horrible. We used extra insecticide, and that caused blistering all over my neck and arms. To control the huge mosquito problem, our officers got some Saudi trucks to spray a pesticide around the area. When they sprayed, I would often develop an incapacitating headache, start vomiting, become dizzy and confused, and end up on the floor. Many times my husband, who was serving in the same unit, asked to take me to a hospital, but his request was denied. Sometimes I would have joint pain, muscle pain, and really bad fatigue for days after they sprayed the pesticide.

By the time we returned to the States, I was getting headaches every time I started my diesel vehicle, but I didn't know what was wrong with me. My husband and I rented an apartment that was literally shiny and new. When we walked into it, I started dry heaving. I became pale and sweaty and was so tired I had to sit down. The guy showing the place to us wanted to call an ambulance, but my husband said, "No, she's OK, this happens all the time." I didn't realize at that point that it was the new paint, new carpets, new cupboards, new vinyl floors, etc., that were bothering me, so we moved into the apartment. After that, I was sick all the time. At work the diesel fumes and cigarette smoke were also making me sick. I was suffering from major depression at this point, but reacted to all the medications that my doctor prescribed.

When President Clinton proposed the early-out program, I took advantage of the opportunity to get out of the military. I decided to join the Reserves so that they would pay for me to attend school to become a licensed practical nurse (LPN). Fortunately, they payed active duty pay so we wouldn't have to work while we were attending classes. It's a good thing because I was fatigued, had migraines very frequently, and had this vague joint and muscle pain that never went away. At least when I became an LPN, I finally had health insurance. No one could figure out what exactly was wrong with me, however. The doctors pretty much said it was depression and stress.

My husband and I decided to buy a house in Nashua, New Hampshire, still not realizing that I had this condition of multiple chemical sensitivity. When we went to a VA office to get a form for our house loan, we walked into a crowded office where lots of people were wearing perfume or aftershave. I became nauseous and developed a headache and worse joint pain; I also became confused. The lady that was helping us with the forms asked my husband what was wrong, and once again, he said, "Oh she's allergic to everything. This happens all the time." She then asked, "Were you in the Gulf War?" When I answered yes, she said I should file a VA claim. When I asked her what that meant, she told me that a lot of vets had come back with these weird symptoms and that the VA should take care of us since we had served our country. She even filled out the form for me so we could just get out of that office full of people wearing scented products. A few months later I got a $3,000 check from the government with no explanation. Later I found out that they had ruled that I was service-connected for sinusitis and migraines. My fatigue, memory problems, and joint and muscle pain were invisible, so I got nothing for those symptoms.

When we bought our house, we still didn't realize that I had multiple chemical sensitivity, so we put in new carpets and an oil burner. I tried to avoid going down in the basement because the oil smell made me feel sick. We did install an all-house exhaust fan, and it helped clear the carpet smells out faster. At this point, I started a college program to get my bachelor's degree and to become an RN, but I kept getting sick in class because of all the perfumes and cologne people were wearing. When I learned how to do research online, I at last found out what I had—multiple chemical sensitivity. During this period, I did learn that when I was able to reduce my exposure to things like fragrances, I felt better, and many of my symptoms improved. Since I liked gardening, I spent a lot of the time outdoors.

I was also learning more on line about Gulf War syndrome at this point and ended up being part of a VA study to see whether people like me who had tested positive for mycoplasma fermentans incognitus would benefit from taking an antibiotic for a year. They put me in a double-blind doxycycline study. Now in the past, I had experienced severe nausea and vomiting every time the VA doctor had put me on doxycycline for a sinus infection. When I started throwing up the first day I took the medication for the study, I realized I must be on the real drug, not the placebo. I took this antibiotic for a year, but it did nothing to help my Gulf War syndrome.[1]

After I graduated from college, I found a job in a nursing home, but I met a lot of resistance there from people who wanted to wear their perfume. After I had to leave work because I was sick several times, which meant someone else had to do my job and theirs too, other staff members at least stopped wearing perfume.

Then a new company took over the nursing home and decided to renovate, which meant painting, laying carpets, etc. The company told me to go on medical leave. I applied for short-term disability, but that was denied on the grounds that chemical sensitivity is a pre-existing condition. So I sued them for worker's comp for the time I was out. They were supposed to rehire me, but when I called on the day the medical leave ended, they said I had no position. I went in and applied for three different positions for which I was qualified. I had worked there for three years, but they would not rehire me. By that point, I was extremely depressed, and my husband had divorced me. The doctor tried almost every type of antidepressant, but I reacted to all of them. Everywhere I applied told me they couldn't accommodate my chemical sensitivity or they just didn't call back. I was considering suicide.

While I was making plans to take my own life, I found a job in a state prison. One problem, however, was that it was full of mold; the floors and walls were being eaten by it. They would just cover the area with a metal plate and wait for the next area to break. It was supposed to have been a temporary building, but the state had run out of money

---

[1] Editor's note: It seems highly likely that it can only have been detrimental to Tara's health to spend a year taking an antibiotic to which she was so allergic that it caused her to vomit the first day she took it. This is yet another example of why it is so important for physicians to recognize the existence of multiple chemical sensitivity. Many other sick veterans participating in this doxycycline study would undoubtedly have reacted adversely to this antibiotic because of their underlying chemical sensitivity. In testimony before Congress, Dr. Claudia Miller, who served as the environmental medical consultant for sick Gulf War veterans in the Houston VA's regional referral center, discussed some of her findings. She stated that "nearly 40 percent reported adverse reactions to medications–all since the Gulf War" (see my book *Gulf War Syndrome: Legacy of a Perfect War*, p. 146).

and just continued using this building. But at least it was a job. Unfortunately, I had the same problems all over again with people wearing perfume. One night they saw me have a reaction to the stripper and floor wax, and they never forgot it.

The prison doctor thought I was faking my problems, which exacerbated my situation. I had to put on a gas mask when one particular nurse who wore a lot of perfume entered the building. The doctor continued to wear her perfume and asked me why I didn't just go on disability. A nursing assistant apologized to me one day because she had forgotten that morning and put some perfume on, but the doctor told her not to apologize for wearing her perfume. This happened right after I had explained to the doctor about my chemical sensitivity, how I had developed it during the Gulf War, and what my symptoms were. Unfortunately in this prison most of the staff were extremely negative and downright mean to one another.

I was recently able to leave the prison job because I at last succeeded in getting a job at a VA nursing home. I hope they will be more willing to accommodate my chemical sensitivity because I want so much to keep working, and I particularly enjoy working with veterans because of my experience in the Gulf War.

Lynn Henderson

FEMA Trailer Exposure

In 2001, I lost everything I owned in a house fire. After that disaster, a relative helped me get a piece of land where I could put a mobile home. I moved into that mobile home in March of 2005, and a few months later Katrina destroyed it. I applied for a FEMA trailer, but I had to wait eighteen months to get it. In the meantime, I lived with relatives.

Life became even more complicated when a cousin whose three little girls I was babysitting died in a car accident in August 2007. I ended up taking those children into the new FEMA trailer I had just received. The youngest was only six months old when these little girls came to live with me. Now they are seventeen months old, three years old, and four years old. My eleven-year-old son is also living with me, and my eighteen-year-old daughter lived with me until she graduated from high school last year. We all lived in that FEMA trailer for six months–from August 2007 until February 2008, when the authorities posted a notice on the door saying the trailer should be tested for formaldehyde. When I had it tested, the results that FEMA sent me in a letter dated May 1, 2008, showed an intermediate high level of formaldehyde–130 parts per billion. The results were accompanied by a letter saying that this level of formaldehyde could cause health problems, particularly for small children and the elderly. That letter ended by saying, "FEMA would like to help relocate you into an apartment or other alternative housing." To my great surprise, the day after I received the letter about the test results I received a second letter from FEMA, this one dated May 8, asking if I would like to buy the trailer for $13,162.

I had never had allergies in my life, but after we moved into the FEMA trailer, I started getting sick. The inside of my nose would itch, and my eyes would itch and water. I would just want to claw my eyes and the inside of my nose. I also started getting more headaches. I had never had many headaches before, never even had to take aspirin before. Now I was having headaches four or five times a week. I also started feeling weak. The three year old especially comes to me and says, "My head is hurting." The baby has had nosebleeds after she has one of her sneezing fits. My eleven-year-old son is constantly blowing his nose now, and he sounds like his whole head is stuffed up. He didn't use to have headaches, but he does now.

Another problem that I started having after we moved into the FEMA trailer is that when I start to make a fist, my hands will hurt. I also am having some pain in the calves of my legs and around my back and my shoulder blades. My lower back hurts all the time now. I had no back problems before I started living in the FEMA trailer. In the last six or eight months, I've started feeling like I'm falling apart. At thirty-seven I'm having problems that a seventy-year-old woman would have.

The three-year-old and the seventeen-month-old baby are now very sensitive to all sorts of scented products. I started noticing that when I would put on body lotion after my shower and then walk by the baby, she would sneeze over and over again until she was out of breath. Then in a minute she would start sneezing again. I can't wear perfume any more because it bothers the little girls so much, and they also react to hair spray and cleaning products I use.

When we received the notice saying that there was a dangerous level of formaldehyde in our FEMA trailer, we moved in with my eighty-eight-year-old grandmother. Now I'm taking care of the three little girls that I hope to adopt, my eleven-year-old son, my grandmother, and an invalid uncle. Given how many people are depending upon me, I'm very concerned about the deterioration in my health since I was exposed to the formaldehyde in the trailer. I work in a sub-type job at a school but have no health insurance. The three little girls I'm raising are on Medicaid, but I can't afford to buy insurance, so that's a huge problem.

Robert Bunker

Exxon Valdez Cleanup Worker

I worked for years in construction—roads, pipelines, the Alaska Railroad, seasonal work. In the off-season, when I wasn't working, I worked with churches and nonprofit groups. I wasn't working in March 1989 because I was waiting for the construction season to start. When the oil spill hit, I went down to Valdez and eventually got hired to do spill work. I worked on a cleanup crew from April to September, and I also went back the second summer. In April 1989, I was one of the first people to hit the dirtiest beaches on Naked Island, which was the island closest to the oil spill. I was right in the thick of it, and it was an ugly mess. At that time, I was forty-five and my health was good, but it seems like I've been sick most of the time since then. I have chronic bronchitis and asthma now, and I didn't have those before the spill.

Most of the time we washed oil off the rocks with high-pressure hoses. Lots of times we steamed rocks, and the oil and steam mixed together. We didn't have respirators, so we were breathing this stuff in. All day long we were wallowing in oil. We were falling down all the time. I screwed up my knees real bad slipping on all those oily rocks, and I still have lots of pain in my knees. It was very bad; the rocks were kind of like bowling balls covered with oil. It was a big slippery mess. After the first few days, I was having nightmares that I was drowning in oil.

I worked one day with a chemical called Inipol. The reason that I didn't work with Inipol after that first day was that someone would normally come around in the morning and bang on our doors. They missed me that second day, so I got out late that day, which is why I only worked one day with Inipol. I'm glad I didn't have to work with Inipol more than that one day because they told us that if it got on your skin, it would go in your bloodstream and cause all sorts of problems. That's why I told my supervisor I didn't want to work around chemicals. There was no way we could really keep those chemicals off our skin.

At first we worked off Navy ships, but after that we slept on big barges, hundreds of people on a barge. We had to travel up to twenty miles in smaller boats to get to the beaches where we worked. I was just exhausted from the long hours we worked— seven days a week, twelve hours a day, sometimes more. And travel time didn't count as part of our twelve-hour shift.

My health problems started after the cleanup. I ignored them for a long time, pretending they didn't exist, that I was just getting older. I had chronic bronchitis and asthma diagnosed in 1999, eight years after my work on the oil spill, but I started having those conditions shortly after the cleanup. I also started having lots of stiffness and pain in my fingers, my hips, my feet, and my neck as well as in my knees, which I injured falling on the oil-covered rocks during the spill cleanup. My whole digestive tract has given me fits since my oil-spill work, and I feel nauseated almost all the time. I have bloating, stomach cramps, just lots of pain and misery from my stomach. I have a lot of problem focusing my eyes now, and I often get very tired and lose my coordination and sense of balance. My dad who is eighty-two is in better health; he has more energy than I do now.

I am pretty sensitive to chemicals now, which makes life difficult. I get bad headaches and real shaky when I'm around gasoline or paint fumes or smoke.

I was working on construction up to February 1999 but finally couldn't do it any longer because my health is so bad at this point. Now I'm a janitor, so I make a lot less money than I did in construction. Even though I'm working only twenty-one hours a week, that leaves me completely exhausted. I'm sure the disinfectants and other cleaning products we use aren't helping my health because I'm so sensitive to chemicals now, but I have to earn a living somehow.

Linda Grommes

Computer Systems Analyst

My wife, Linda, was born in Lakeview, Michigan, in 1952, and she graduated as valedictorian of her high school class in 1971 with a perfect 4.0 GPA. Just three years later she received a B.S. degree in Computer Science from Central Michigan University, again with a perfect GPA.

Linda was not a sickly child, and there was nothing that seemed to foreshadow what her life would later become. She was hired by Upjohn as a computer systems analyst, a job that she loved and distinguished herself at. In 1975, having barely launched a promising career and having been married less than a year, she came down with an intense flu-like illness that would not go away. For six months, swelling from throat inflammation would sometimes almost shut down her airways. Her tonsils ulcerated and fever ravaged her, but doctor after doctor assured her that her illness would all be over in a week or two.

When Linda finally recovered—after a fashion—she returned to work, only to relapse a few weeks later. It was like that for years: a few weeks of being "well" enough to drag herself to work followed by a few weeks in bed, over and over.

When I recently met Linda's boss from those days, he told me that Linda was the first person in the history of Upjohn to do something that was unheard of in those days. The company paid several thousand dollars to run a dedicated phone line to her home and gave her a time-sharing terminal so she would not have to come in to work. It was telecommuting before there was a word for it. "Linda accomplished more in a half day than some of the other people in her group did in a whole week," her former boss said. "It was a no-brainer decision to keep her working as long as possible."

Eventually, Linda was given a diagnosis of chronic fatigue syndrome (CFS). Then at a later point she was given a diagnosis of myalgic encephalomyelitis (ME), the term used in the European Union for particularly serious cases of unrelenting fatigue and recurring fever like

Linda's. Her deteriorating cognitive abilities eventually forced her onto disability, which she received on the basis of a measured drop in IQ from 180 to 102 over a two-year period.

Characteristically, despite this staggering loss, Linda simply re-invented herself. She had grown up on a dairy farm and had always had a special relationship with animals. She became a gifted breeder and trainer of Shetland sheepdogs ("Shelties") and raised several who became U.S. and Canadian champions. Her top champion, Chris, graces the cover of one of the popular Sheltie books to this day.

Linda established Dayspring Kennels at a beautiful farm in Allegan, Michigan, and branched out into Shetland sheep—after all, that is what Shelties were bred to herd. Because of the delays and hassle of dealing with the Shetland sheep registry in the U.K., she founded a registry for North America that eventually grew into the North American Shetland Sheep Association.

Unfortunately, deteriorating health and the end of her first marriage forced Linda to sell her beloved farm and nearly all her animals. She moved to Kalamazoo, Michigan, with her retired champions Chris and Sonny to figure out what awaited her next.

That's when Linda came into my life. Neither of us exactly believed the ensuing whirlwind courtship; we were married in 1994, less than six months after we had met. It wasn't really either of our styles, but in retrospect, I am eternally grateful for all the living and loving we packed into the next six years.

Those familiar with the "push/crash" phenomenon in chronic fatigue syndrome know that the only way for someone with that illness to do "normal" things is to "push through" for however many hours or days they can and then "pay the price," often being bed-bound for some weeks thereafter. This was the only way Linda was able to realize her love of travel and other activities that I had the honor of sharing with her. We made it all the way to London in the late spring of 2000, but it was even more difficult than usual because Linda was increasingly sensitive to the perfumes, fragrances, and petrochemical fumes involved in such a trip.

Over the next three years or so, it became obvious to us that Linda's life was shrinking still further, and probably for good. Fortunately her physician, a specialist in chronic illness, was as familiar with MCS as he was with chronic fatigue syndrome, and he recognized her chemical sensitivity immediately.

One of the largest problems for Linda was that she became acutely sensitive to the mycotoxins given off by mold during this period. Living as we did in a desert in Arizona, mold was not nearly the problem it would have been in other climates, but Linda had a lot of books, papers, award certificates, and the like from her years in Michigan that had originally resided in a moldy basement back on her farm. By disposing of all these treasures, most of our books, and replacing all the carpeting in the house with tile, we were able to pretty much eliminate mold as an issue in our home environment, but by then the damage had already been done.

Linda became sensitive to the slightest amounts of volatile organic chemicals (VOCs) to the point that she was unable to leave the house, except to see a doctor. Even that excursion out of her controlled environment usually produced more harm than any help the medical appointment could yield.

Many aspects of daily life became a struggle. For example, the neighbors on one side used fabric softener copiously, filling our backyard with clouds of strong-smelling fumes whenever they ran their dryer, which was frequently. For this and other reasons, it was very risky for us to leave the windows open for fresh air or for Linda to venture outside in the sun to enjoy the lush backyard whose landscaping she had designed and nurtured.

Because of neurological problems, Linda could no longer stand to watch videos and could not read more than a paragraph or two at a time. No more books, virtually no form of mental escape from the daily torment. Linda said that she would not wish this disease on her worst enemy, a sentiment I've heard from more than one MCS patient.

No disease is a respecter of persons, but there seemed to be something particularly awful about the combination of Linda and MCS. Linda loved and relished life in an extraordinary way; MCS brought her every imaginable form of death. She had experienced a lot of physical suffering in life with dignity and grace; MCS raised that suffering to unimaginable levels. She was the antithesis of the self-centered drama queen, yet MCS put her in the middle of crisis after humiliating crisis and rendered her helpless. Linda was all about transcending her limitations, but MCS required her to adopt an ever-vigilant stance to protect herself from the everyday trappings of life that she used to embrace with enthusiasm. She had been a powerful, strong, intelligent woman; MCS reduced her to a confused wreck who at times could not remember my name.

I find it difficult to describe my feelings about what I witnessed happening to Linda at the day-by-day, minute-by-minute level that no one else saw. In its worst forms, MCS seems to be designed by hell itself to destroy a person at the most fundamental level. It is not simply a mindless tumor crowding out healthy tissue; it is not simply a fact of biology compromising one's bodily functions. There were times in Linda's case when MCS seemed to me like a malevolent intelligence bent not just on taking life but on exacting the maximum possible mental, emotional, spiritual, and physical suffering.

The whole experience did far more to undermine my faith, however, than it did Linda's. Sure, Linda had tears of loss and frustration, but she never stopped believing that there was some kind of overarching reason and purpose for even what her life had become. "God is there in the really big, important crossroads," she was fond of saying. She believed he would provide for her at that moment when she left this world for whatever comes next.

Somehow she was still able to tell her family, "I've had a good life." Somehow in her final months she worked hard to pull together a life scrapbook and to write a barely legible but heartfelt personal note to each and every one of her loved ones and closest friends. Somehow she chose a simple bequest for each person and saw to it that I packed them in a box and that it was all noted down on a checklist so that I would be sure these things got to the right people despite the chaos and grief right after her death.

When she finished these tasks in late June of this year, it was down to a simple waiting game. "I might last another year," she said, "but sometimes it seems like there can't be more than a few days left in me."

We lay on our bed the Sunday before she died, watching a gentle and much-needed rain fall on the desert vista outside the window. "It's so beautiful," she said softly, struggling to focus, a little echo of the awe and wonder coming back to her voice for a few seconds. "I have gotten to see so much beauty."

One morning I had gotten up early, leaving Linda to sleep. She had been up off and on all night as usual and had changed her nightshirt

three times because of the massive sweats she had pretty much continuously. These night sweats had apparently become her body's main
method of getting rid of toxins. I did a little work and went to have
coffee with some friends. When I came back, Linda was gone, and I was
grateful that her end appeared to have been peaceful. She was only fifty-
four.

I am not sure what happened to the rest of that day. The authorities
asked questions, and as is always the case when someone dies at home,
gathered evidence and took her body off for autopsy. I won't know for
months, I'm told, an official cause of death, but the details are not a
matter of much curiosity to me, other than to know it wasn't agonizing
for her. And as agonizing as her life had become, even that wouldn't
bother me as much as one might think. Linda had said to me some
weeks earlier that she felt now she could bear anything as long as she
knew it wasn't going to last too long.

Perhaps in death, as in life, the medical professionals will not know
the right questions to ask or how to recognize what is in front of them
to see. I'm certain of this much: the cause of Linda's death will be listed
as anything other than "multiple chemical sensitivity." The disease will
be invisible to the end. "MCS," they'll say to themselves, "doesn't kill
people. We're not even sure it exists." Linda and I know better.

Jill Sverdlove

9/11 Exposure

In the fall of 2001, at the age of thirty-two, my life was full. I'd worked hard in my career and was the president of a thriving business in New York City. I spent long hours in the office and nights and weekends with friends–dancing, attending concerts, restaurants, readings, or movies. I dated musicians, practiced yoga, and threw great parties in my Upper West Side brownstone. Although I was enjoying my life, I looked forward to marriage, kids, and owning a home someday soon.

Within two years, my health, work, apartment, friends, car, and all my belongings would vanish. I would be surviving one fragrance-free breath at a time.

*　*　*　*　*

Three days after September 11, 2001, I began to have what I now call "reactions" to my office. I had no idea at first that something had started to happen to my body. The onset of illness began so gradually that it would take two more years and a final debilitating exposure before I would be diagnosed properly. It would take much longer before I understood the full story.

I started my morning on September 11, 2001, by heading to a meeting downtown. As I was leaving my apartment, my roommate exclaimed something about a plane and the World Trade Center. I thought nothing of it, worrying instead that I would be late for my appointment if I didn't hurry.

Soon after I boarded my subway train, it was abruptly halted in a dark tunnel between stops. We remained stuck in the subway system for an inordinately long time, hearing only the muffled sounds of the conductor attempting communication. Our silence indicated we all sensed the same thing: something was very wrong, more than the average-day-in-NYC wrong. Later I would learn that not far from where we were trapped in our subway train, the Twin Towers had started to collapse, people were jumping off the falling buildings, and Lower

Manhattan was filled with thick smoke and debris. By the time we finally escaped from our subway car by working our way through an underground maze of pungent tunnels, the world outside was surreal–clouds of dense black and green and gray smoke billowing beneath a clear, cloudless sky. That day, and for a long time afterwards, the sky would remain full of soot and chemicals. Like many others, after I reached my office, I soon headed down the West Side, back toward Ground Zero, wanting to understand what had happened, wanting to see something tangible.

A few days later, when I was back at work in my office on Columbus Circle, I noticed that even though our offices were on the eighth floor, I could smell the fumes from the truck filling the petroleum tank in the basement, although I had previously never noticed these fumes. The kitchen smoke from the restaurant on the ground floor of our building also suddenly began to severely irritate me. And something in my private office was causing me to have severe headaches, even though I'd never had headaches like these prior to 9/11.

When I spent time in my office, my brain felt swollen and heavy and my fingers became hot, red, and tingly. My eyes burned, and my throat felt sore and scratchy. At that stage, since I mostly noticed major sensations in my office, I was convinced something in that room was causing the reactions. But there was no World Trade Center dust inside my office because it was so far from Ground Zero, so there was nothing obvious to clean.

Days and then weeks passed. Soon I noticed that even the larger area around my private office set off physical problems. The copy machine induced dizziness and nausea, the fax made me loopy. Standing near my moldy air conditioning unit, even when it was off, wiped me out. When I was working on my computer, I experienced viselike headaches and, what was strangest for me, a fogginess in my brain that left me feeling extremely spacey.

I went to a doctor who assured me that I had no "regular" allergies and suggested that perhaps all I needed was an air filter for the office. Although the office air had never been great (it was an old building), I didn't understand how it suddenly could be affecting me in any way. I wouldn't learn for years that the 9/11 toxic exposures had initiated a sensitivity to chemicals and to the mycotoxins given off by molds. (The air conditioner and carpet harbored molds, and the office machines gave

off chemicals.) Back then I had no idea what volatile organic compounds were, nor could I fathom the connection between air quality and
my symptoms. I was a longtime runner. I was a New Yorker. I survived
on bad air. But I followed the doctor's advice and bought a mega HEPA
air filter for the office anyway.

It didn't make the slightest difference.

*   *   *   *   *

Prior to September 11, I had been in pretty decent overall health. I'd had
some recent foot surgeries, an appendectomy, and a few health problems
like hypothyroidism, for which I took medication. I had been a distance
runner for years, only recently stopping because of foot problems. After
I had to give up running, I took up yoga. My life was about movement,
and I rarely sat still, instead always working, exercising, playing.

As the president of Gotham Writers' Workshop, the largest creative
writing school in the country, it was my job to manage all aspects of the
company, from finances and marketing to future planning. I dealt with
80 employees and 6,000 students a year. The two original founders were
full-time writers who were absentee owners, so almost all responsibility
fell to me. During the six years I ran the business, I had taken a small,
fledgling workshop and grown it into a successful multimillion-dollar
business. At that point, it was my priority, and I loved it. The last thing
I wanted to do was tell my bosses that I was having strange reactions to
certain objects in the office, maybe even to the office itself. Besides, I
wasn't debilitated, and my reactions were still manageable.

However, over the next few weeks, along with the occasional
tingling in my limbs and the thick head pain, I couldn't fend off the odd
sense that I was slowly deteriorating.

When I was at home in my Upper West Side apartment, I would feel
normal, which kept my concern in balance. And yet each morning, after
only a short time in the office, the headaches and pain would come
back. Nonetheless, I continued functioning at high levels despite a sense
that my health was slipping away.

Then other incidents occurred. I had been attempting to buy an
apartment. A few places I looked at caused me to experience the same
awful sensations I suffered in the office. Then I had a bad reaction in a
friend's car in which the carpeting had become moldy as the result of a

water leak from a broken window. After being in the car for a half hour, I passed out. Although I rationalized that these events were brief and the problem was primarily just in my office, the urge to escape the city began to take hold, and I stopped apartment hunting.

More physical issues were brewing. My hormone and thyroid levels went awry again after having been stable for years. I had strange aches, especially in my lower right abdomen after eating. My sinuses were so occluded that people often mistakenly thought I had a cold. As my viselike headaches continued, I decided to tell the owners that something was wrong, and I asked for a different office.

But the owners were rarely in the facility, had little understanding of my situation, and were opposed to spending money on another office (even though we were bursting at the seams). After some tension, they eventually compromised, and I rented another room on a different floor in the same building for me and the two other employees. I felt noticeably better there. Unfortunately, my bosses only temporarily appeased me. Even though they had previously deemed my performance exceptional and I had brought in significant profits over the years, they were worried about the welfare of the company. I was worried about my welfare. The situation was becoming very uncomfortable.

The longing to leave New York became a scorching thirst, my body screaming "Get Out." In the fall of 2002, I gave up my rights in the company, negotiated a deal that provided me enough funds to get by for a short while, and fled New York, believing all would then be fine.

Back then, I didn't know I was showing signs of chemical sensitivity. I had never even heard of it, nor had anyone around me. I can only wonder what would have happened if someone had recognized the onset and explained what was going on in my body before it got worse, but the reality is that most of us don't learn until it's too late.[1]

*　　*　　*　　*　　*

---

[1] Editor's note: A few months after 9/11, my Chemical Sensitivity Foundation ran several ads in a free newspaper that distributes 10,000 copies near Ground Zero. We hoped to alert New Yorkers to the possibility that they might develop chemical sensitivity from their exposure to the WTC toxins, but at this point, few were ready to hear that message.

After I left New York, I went to Virginia Beach, Virginia, to regroup while helping a girlfriend with her business there. A mutual friend offered a rental that her husband had recently purchased for only $20,000, an old house built in 1923. The moment I walked inside I got a bad headache. "It smells strange in here," I told my friend, but she convinced me that the odor was from a floor cleaner. I didn't want to appear ungrateful, so I moved in.

Only later would I learn that the attic had a leaking water tank and the damp insulation up there was covered in very visible mold. The previous tenant had even encouraged the moisture in order to grow marijuana in the attic, as the remnants attested. All this directly over my bedroom.

Within weeks, especially when I was inside the house, I started having blinding headaches that drained me of all energy. My sinuses throbbed with pain, and every morning I woke up with uncomfortably swollen hands and incredible fatigue. My digestion deteriorated, causing me to lose weight rapidly.

But when I complained to my friend about the mold in the house, which was visible in some places and reeked all over, she and her husband just laughed. "Mold is everywhere," they told me. "You just have an allergy. Everyone has allergies."

I scrubbed the house with bleach and a powerful chemical spray that my friend's husband provided. The smell and my reactions worsened, and my breathing problems progressed to the point that I needed medical attention and eventually an inhaler. I had never had asthma before, nor such intense lung pain.

Six months too late I would discover that the old house had extremely high levels of toxic black molds: Stachybotrous, Aspergillus, Penicillium, and more. I would also eventually discover how dangerous black mold and the mycotoxins they give off are, especially for someone like me, who had already started to develop chemical sensitivity.

The hit to my already susceptible system was too much. I naively downed antibiotics as my list of symptoms now included huge hives, unrelenting diarrhea, Candida with yeast infections, a chronic sinus infection, and a head thick with a brain fog that wouldn't lift until I was out of the house for hours.

I finally decided to leave, taking my clothes, journals, pictures, computer, and furniture out of the Virginia house and moving it all into my parents' suburban New York home. Unfortunately, within a few days I realized all my belongings I had brought along smelled horrible. The stench was unmistakable–a slightly sweet yet pungent smell, just like the odor inside the Virginia rental house. Although there is no feasible way to get rid of mycotoxins, my mom and I didn't realize this and were convinced we could fix the problem. First, my mother took me to a doctor, who put me on Prednisone. (I later learned that, like anti-biotics, this steroid destroys good bacteria in the gut and ultimately feeds fungus even more.) Then we began a major cleaning operation. I sniffed each item (a.k.a. inhaling fungal spores into my sinus tissue) to check what stank (everything did). We laundered, bleached, and dry-cleaned clothing. Finally, we sprayed and scrubbed all other items, walls, and floors with disinfectant and other heavy-duty chemicals.

The next morning the Jill I knew was gone. I had disappeared into an endless reaction, unable to breathe, function, think clearly, sleep, or hold any food in. I had started to react to everything. Re-exposure to the cleaners we had just used made my throat close up. The computer made my hands sting, and the cell phone made my head feel as if it was being crushed. My clothes gave me hives, and an incessant throbbing pain took hold in my left sinus and never let up for the next three years. Experiencing an endless massive reaction, I was convinced this meant the mold had gotten onto everything.

We didn't realize then that I was reacting to more than the mold. I was also reacting to extremely low levels of fragrances and other chemicals, like those in the cleaning products we were using. My 9/11 toxic exposures had triggered multiple chemical sensitivity (MCS), and then the subsequent mold exposure in Virginia, the steroids, and our massive cleaning project had finally pushed me into an extreme case of chemical sensitivity and electromagnetic sensitivity. Furthermore, the allergists I saw were not trained to recognize or treat the effects of chemical injury, as MCS is a response to toxic exposures, not an allergic reaction.

I could think of no other solution but to move again, and Boulder, Colorado, seemed an appealing destination. I had discovered Boulder on a cross-country trip after college and had lived there for eight months. Now I felt the urge to return, my body craving the mountain air.

By this point, my mom and I had learned from professional industrial hygienists that, sure enough, I had brought the dangerous molds from the Virginia house into my mom's attic, my bedroom, and her basement, contaminating everything in those rooms. Eventually I was also tested and showed exorbitantly high, off-the-chart levels of exposure, especially to Stachybotrous mold mycotoxins (one of the most dangerous toxic molds). The toxicologists told me to get rid of everything, including my cat, Angus, who was also showing signs of mycotoxin poisoning from the Virginia rental.

But it's not easy throwing out all that you own. I loved my cat, and my identity was still attached to my belongings. My stuff would be fine, I reasoned, if it was cleaned enough and aired out. I would heal and my cat would too. I just had to leave.

And so, dressed in clothing that still contained some residues of mold and fabric softener, I donned a face mask (to the surprise of many interstate truckers) and drove off in my mycotoxin-marinated Celica convertible, my kitty and all my contaminated belongings in tow. At that point, the idea of mycotoxin poisoning was so surreal to me and so hard to accept that I even paid movers a few thousand dollars to truck the rest of my smelly stuff out to Colorado.

When the movers arrived in Boulder, I suffered an anaphylactic reaction to the mycotoxins in my belongings. Despite endless cleanings, my old stuff contaminated my new rental and ruined a few more rentals after that. A lot of lessons had to be learned, time had to pass, and most of my savings had to be lost before my stubbornness subsided and I realized that the mycotoxins given off by toxic mold can't be eliminated by cleaning and they don't disappear over time. I would never again tolerate my stuff, not even my car, not even in Colorado. Any proximity to my belongings induced hives, shooting pains up my arms, diarrhea, a band of strange pressure pushing down on my eyebrows and into my temples, and mental reactions that ranged from irritability to paranoia.

A year later, when my urine tested positive for continued exposure to high levels of Stachybotrous mycotoxins, I finally knew I could no longer keep hauling my belongings around with me. They all had to go: the sexy, one-of-a-kind New York City clothes, my cozy old sweaters, my antique bookshelf and other furniture, my Trek mountain bike, my cherished lifetime collection of books, my files and letters and correspondence of thirty-five years, my grandma's jewelry box and my dad's family paintings. An endless list of loss from memory chatchkas and hand drums to hundreds of personally designed baseball caps from the hat company I had run before moving to Gotham Writers' Workshop. Even my beloved convertible car was still contaminated, and it too had to go.

Most heartbreaking of all was giving up my cat and best friend of ten years. With treatment, Angus had recovered fairly well from the mold exposure, but I could no longer care for him. In tears, I took him to a friend's place.

It would have been easier to convince myself that this was all psychological, but the reality was that the experiment could be duplicated. Whenever I was exposed to these mycotoxin-contaminated items (which still smelled so much that others noticed the odor), I reacted severely. If that wasn't convincing enough, even without knowing the history, others with sensitivities also reacted to my stuff.

Finally all that was left of my former life was a big plastic tub with a lifetime of journals and pictures wrapped in dozens of Ziplocs and Hefty bags. I could never again open that sealed sarcophagus without severe physical repercussions.

Unfortunately, although I felt significantly better after getting rid of my contaminated belongings, the fuzzy brain fog remained with me, as did my extreme sensitivity to synthetic fragrances and other chemicals. When I was reacting to an exposure, besides intense physical and emotional responses, I would sometimes lose the ability to speak properly, to write, spell, remember things, or have word recall.

By this point, I no longer tolerated any house or apartment because of my hypersensitivity to so many things found in indoor environments. Gas heat depleted me. Washers and dryers in which conventional detergents had been used were unbearable. Scented candles and plug-in air fresheners crippled my digestion and made me feel irrationally violent. There were many other triggers: gas stoves, formaldehyde (in carpet, most cabinets, and new paint), pesticides, flame-retardant-covered mattresses, and fabric softener used by roommates or wafting from neighbors' dryer vents. Any place near major roads proved problematic because I reacted to the auto and diesel exhaust wafting through the windows. Old places meant mold, and new ones meant formaldehyde. My reactions were endless and sounded ludicrous to real estate agents and potential housemates.

People with chemical sensitivity usually develop new food intolerances, and I was no exception, so my digestion was shot by this point. I appeared gaunt and pale, my eyes sunken and underlined with black circles. Although I was exhausted, I had great difficulty sleeping. My throat was raw and hoarse from continual exposures, the throbbing in my sinuses beat on, and my hair started falling out in clumps.

At last, I found a doctor who diagnosed me as having MCS, which she only knew about because she, too, suffered from it. Then I learned about a book that clarified everything that had happened to me: *"Multiple Chemical Sensitivity: A Survival Guide,"* by Pamela Reed Gibson. This book was an immense help to me as I made decisions about how to live with MCS.

During that spring and summer of 2003, I spent most of my time outdoors, living and camping high in the mountains near Edwards, Colorado, where a friend lived. My goal was to spend as much time as possible outside in the fresh air, clearing my lungs and sweating out toxins.

Any attempt to live a normal life backfired. I stubbornly tried to go into a beauty salon to get my hair cut (and, crazy as it sounds, dyed, because it was coming in all gray). As soon as the dye was brought out, my nose started to bleed and I had shooting pains throughout my limbs. Although I quickly left, I developed an incapacitating headache that lasted for days.

I also attempted to work in a small mountain bookstore. That was a terrible idea because the printer's ink on the books and the perfume on the tourists sent me spiraling still lower. I made a few new friends, and even tried having a relationship, but my strange situation was hard for anyone to understand and hard enough for me to deal with.

Trying to reach out to former friends proved futile. With MCS, there is continual stress not only from loss, lack of control, homelessness, uncertainty, misdiagnosis, and physical pain, but also from the constant skepticism of others. Perhaps the most devastating aspect, unique to this illness, was the lack of support from friends. Hardly anyone understands MCS. Most people don't know how to deal with this illness, nor do they want to. It's too overwhelming to think that common, everyday chemicals can affect some people in such an extreme way. The issue is compounded by the fact that chemical companies have immense power and want to make MCS sound controversial.

Calling friends for support had become difficult. Most could not empathize, and I knew they were thinking, "You're a New Yorker who flipped her lid. No one is allergic to the world, and I'm sorry, but unless you can talk about a good new restaurant in SoHo or Brooklyn real estate there's really nothing left to this relationship." Although my mother remained supportive, my brother and sister were busy with their kids and couldn't comprehend my condition. And the Virginia friend whose husband owned the rented moldy house also conveniently disappeared from my life, not wanting to hear how sick I'd become.

The loneliness of this condition caused me incredible heartache. But knowing that stress is one of many causes and effects of illness, I realized I would have to minimize it in order to heal. I could no longer waste energy asking for understanding and help from others, nor try to change their beliefs. And trying to defend my sanity only made me seem more insane. I wouldn't bother anymore.

There were many times when I thought death would be easier, especially when I was having a bad reaction. My life and my purpose felt so diminished, and I was beyond exhausted. Somehow survival instinct propelled me forward, however, and I researched and networked until I found a decent Colorado environmental illness specialist who confirmed the MCS diagnosis and was familiar with treatments for some of my symptoms. He put me through ten weeks of hyperbaric oxygen chamber therapy, which improved my brain function noticeably.

I believe it was the mountains, though, that probably saved my life. The fresh air helped sooth my damaged lungs, and the tranquility and clarity of nature maintained my sanity. Daily yoga played a big role, too. But as winter approached, the cold was pushing me indoors, and I decided to move down to Boulder, which was on the edge of the plains and much more temperate. It was also full of health food stores and open-minded people.

The endless home search continued to be futile, as my notebooks filled with scribbled addresses and tiny pull tabs from bulletin board flyers. Many nights I slept on strangers' floors to test potential places, thereby creating interesting memories and even friendships. At last, I found a room I tolerated in a huge historical landmark house full of all-natural students from Naropa, a Buddhist college. Although I often slept on the porch, at least I could rest without inhaling unrelenting synthetic fragrances.

Unfortunately, I soon could no longer tolerate this house, and I had problems with the other places that I tried, for various reasons from roommates' fragranced products to renovations. In the meantime, I went to dozens of practitioners, trying everything, squandering my savings in the desperate hope that some healer's promised cure would solve my problems. Some poked me with needles to draw blood or move qi. Others caked me in clay, soaked my feet in rust colored water, and irrigated my colon. I went on the Blood Type Diet, the Maker's Diet, the Candida Diet, and the 28-Day Cleanse. All that became clear was I felt better when I was away from chemical exposures.

By the spring of 2004, I was worn out, yet still felt driven to find a solution to this nightmare. I had lost my belongings three more times because they had been contaminated by chemical or mold exposures. I had lost my sense of identity and no longer even had my pictures or journals to conjure up memories of my past. My passions went neglected because I was unable to read or write anymore. In the mirror, I saw a pale and puffy-faced stranger with one eye drooping and a thin mess of dried frizz that had once been my curly mane of pride. I needed help.

Unexpectedly, at this time my nonsmoking stepfather was diagnosed with lung cancer. Armed with oxygen and a respirator, I made it back to New York just in time to visit with my ailing stepdad, now hairless and hollow-eyed. Although he had never before been expressive, he hugged me close and told me he finally understood my situation. My parents decided to send me to a renowned environmental health clinic in Dallas, Texas. He died the day after I left for the clinic.

The clinic didn't produce a miracle, but it did provide validation and support, especially from the hundreds of other patients who were experiencing the same thing. There were Gulf War veterans, nurses, teachers, pilots, executives, artists, and more, all poisoned by pesticides, formaldehyde, disinfectant, mercury, black mold, burning oil fields, or other toxins. One investment banker's health had crashed after exposure to air fresheners.

Multiple medical tests, a neuropsychological evaluation, brain scans and skin injections, all for measuring toxic injury, provided further tangible proof that my chemical sensitivity was a serious problem. I was diagnosed with toxic encephalopathy, peripheral neuropathy, vasculitis, chronic inflammation, toxic exposure to specific heavy metals and mycotoxins, severe hypothyroid, digestive disorders, impaired detoxification, gluten intolerance, autonomic nervous system dysfunction, chronic sinusitis, allergic food gastroenteritis, immune dysfunction, chemical sensitivity, and more.

I learned that exposures could make my emotional state feel like an out-of-body experience because the nasal passage connects directly through the blood-brain-barrier to our limbic lobe, which controls our most basic emotions like fear, anger, and elation. So inhaling a synthetic fragrance can immediately cause neurological changes that can affect everything from memory evocation to mood, an effect that is magnified for people with MCS.

After spending a few months in Texas, I returned to Boulder, continuing the detoxification protocol locally with daily saunas, shots, supplements, oxygen, and biweekly IVs. I also resumed the search for a safe home. But I remained nomadic–house, tent, and car hopping, fleeing in the middle of the night from mosquito spraying, fragrance emitted by neighbors' dryers, or cigarette smoke.

But camping proved a blessing. One weekend I set up my tent near an outdoor bluegrass festival (many passions had to go, but not music if I could help it). While I was standing there, drenched in the pouring rain, a beautiful green-eyed man walked up to me and asked, "Would you like to share my umbrella?" After momentarily debating the risk of detergent on his clothing, I agreed. After all, it was my thirty-sixth birthday, why not be daring? Matthew is still with me, and I've never loved a better man.

After Matthew made the switch to safer products and turned off the gas heat in his condo, I was even able to tolerate his place for a while. ("Hi, I'll be your girlfriend, but I'm homeless. Do you mind if I move in?") Then his neighbor plugged in four air fresheners, and fumes seeped into Matthew's condo, triggering in me a bloody nose, vomiting, and an irrational anger towards Matthew. Thankfully, he was familiar with my reactions by then and tolerated them (and my incessant sniffing of his clothes and hair).

The air freshener fumes, however, clung to the walls of Matthew's condo, and I was homeless again. There I was at age thirty-seven brushing my teeth in the local co-op restroom, bathing in Boulder Creek, and sleeping everywhere, when in a parallel life I might have been a suburban mom shepherding her kids to school in her big SUV.

And then finally, after three years of checking out an enormous number of places to buy or rent (I couldn't afford, or chance, trying to build a new safe house), my luck changed. An unscented acquaintance put her off-gassed, 1970s apartment on the market. After sleeping there for a while to test the place out, in October of 2005, at long last, I bought a safe apartment.

During the next year, I experienced a great deal of relief in my safe apartment, where double weather stripping and enormous air filters helped block outside fumes. I also bought safe detergent and fabric softener for my neighbors and convinced my homeowners' association to use organic lawn care. I added a filter to every faucet and used electric appliances and electric baseboard heat. I slept on an organic, flame-retardant-free mattress. A space-age-looking vapor barrier (Denny foil) covered the concrete subfloor that remained after I tore out the carpet. My mother helped by buying me a small infrared sauna where I sweat daily to help eliminate toxins.

Something changed though, and during the summer of 2006, despite all my precautions, the apartment picked up some sort of contamination that I couldn't tolerate. A neighbor's renovations? A faulty washing machine issue? In trying to salvage the place, I ripped it apart. Finally, after sleeping on the deck for months while attempting every solution and praying the problem would resolve itself, I moved out. With no other options, even though I still didn't do well at Matthew's place with the lingering fruity fragrance from his neighbor's air fresheners, I once again moved in with him, this time bringing portable oxygen and six air filters.

*   *   *   *   *

So this is my life now in 2006:

I've learned to live with many unimaginable limitations and must always be prepared to leave a situation when chemical exposures occur. I try not to get attached to places, clothes, furniture, or cars. (I've gone through five cars in four years. The last one leaked antifreeze.) Now I drive a dented, paint-peeling, 1992 Chrysler LeBaron with the carpet ripped out–a symbolic change from the cute Celica Convertible with which I began this journey.)

Exposures abound, and I can't be in most public places or stores or even near houses spewing fabric softener from dryer vents without feeling awful. Even though I often wear a mask, which still embarrasses me, I have problems in these places. Overall, I remain ceaselessly on guard, knowing too well that my health could suddenly deteriorate again because of one more bad exposure, like when they start spraying pesticides in the spring.

My social life is obviously limited. Nearly every store, home, office, and public bathroom contains air fresheners. Besides a lack of places I can go to, friends are loaded with fragranced products and most would rather not change their shampoo for me.

I find balance through spending a lot of time in nature, embracing the part of life I can still enjoy. Despite a bad foot, I often navigate the mountain trails around Boulder (albeit holding my breath when detergent-scented hikers pass). Matthew and I spend most weekends camping, or in our organic community garden plot. Although I am legally disabled and surviving on Social Security disability income, I volunteer for short periods at the local co-op, spend a lot of time helping others who are newly tripping into MCS, and devote much passion to my newfound armchair activism, like fighting pesticide use and corrupt trade secret laws for synthetic fragrances. But I still dream about the next venture I will start someday when the business of health isn't so all encompassing.

Sometimes the things I miss overwhelm me. I long to go to concerts, yoga classes, a friend's party, or even to pump my own gas. I ache to travel, and I miss working, which is impossible because I cannot be in offices or use a computer for any length of time without having a reaction. Ultimately, I'm learning how to do less.

While I try to maintain peace within, without a safe home, there is still a sense of urgency as Matthew and I watch my health slide instead of stabilize as it had been doing before. When I lived in my formerly tolerated apartment and was following a careful diet and utilizing daily oxygen and a sauna, I was functioning at a higher level. My brain came back 100 percent. I could go into some stores. I was able to use a computer again (with the CPU in the closet) for about two hours before my hands and head would tingle and swell. My emotions and hormones stabilized. I could read new books that had baked in the sun for a few weeks. And I was writing again. Although I wasn't cured, I felt dramatic improvement in my symptoms, and the experience taught Matthew and me that avoidance of chemical exposures through having a safe home, coupled with ongoing treatments, are key to my having some level of normalcy with MCS.

Now we are searching for land, which is rare and exorbitantly expensive in Boulder, but after checking out a huge number of existing houses, we believe we have no other choice than to build a nontoxic home in the mountains. We've also witnessed people I've met with MCS function much better when they moved into homes they had specially built. So we search, and we hope, and we wait, trying not to worry about where the money will come from or what would happen if we spent everything building and it didn't work for me. Instead we drive around and fantasize about the healthy home we'll enjoy one day, about the kids we'll be able to have, about what it would be like to be able to open up our windows and breathe fresh air.

I used to believe in a magic-bullet cure, and I tried all the treatments that promised such a dream. Today, while I can't bury that unfounded hope entirely, I have a deeper understanding of how this condition works, and so I put my energy instead toward finding a way to manage my symptoms, creating a safe space, helping others through this, and finding joy in the smallest of moments. Although I keep researching new theories and treatments diligently, I know that for me avoidance is the best way to live symptom free because when I am not around any irritants, I feel strong, sane, and clear-headed.

I have bounced around all the emotional phases of illness. I've gone through the stage of feeling enormous regrets, of attempting to justify why I should be sick now. I've experienced rage and depression, bitterness, hope, and acceptance. And I know my situation can and will change all over again.

Now, although I have mourned the loss, it seems useless to wonder what my life would be like if I had never been exposed to the 9/11 toxins and then the mold in the old house in Virginia. Instead, the enormous challenge lies in creating a new sense of purpose. In the past, so much of my identity was tied with my career. But today I am only just beginning to understand how all that has happened to me matters only in who I become. To me, this means having better, healthier priorities–focusing on treating myself, others, and the environment well, following my passions, and loving deeply, while also being careful not to tie my identity only to my disability.

I've also had to accept how vulnerable we all are. And while there may be reasons I'm more susceptible than others, the reality is that these toxins can affect anyone. To that end, I hope there is purpose and meaning in telling my story and that my doing so may help keep someone else from going down the path to chronic illness.

Epilogue:

It is now August, 2008. Matthew and I are married and on April 16, I gave birth to our beautiful baby girl, Isabel. Although she has digestive issues and allergies to foods I eat (I'm breastfeeding after years of detoxing), she is otherwise happy and healthy. The pregnancy and labor were extremely difficult with complications, but Isabel is well worth it.

We also just broke ground on our healthy house in the foothills of Boulder.

Having a loving partner and an amazing daughter has brought such meaning and joy to my life. Every day, however, I remain challenged by MCS issues.

Sfc. Roy Twymon

Gulf War Veteran

From the time we was given the PB pill, we was told to continue to take them. We kept on taking them, and we kept on taking them till after the war. And I noticed then that I started having diarrhea, my bowel was a different color. I had to run to the outdoor toilet because sometime, you know, it be that severe, the diarrhea.

The night prior to going into Iraq the wind was blowing our direction while they was bombing. And I had respiratory problems that night and some more personnel did also. When we got up in Iraq, going down the highway we saw bodies everywhere lying, bodies stuck to the steering wheel, bodies lying on the floor, on the ground, vehicles burning where they had bombed the vehicle with these shells, and, you know, all this smoke and everything. And then we finally set up camp right next to these bunkers everybody had been talking about. They was blowing up bunkers practically every day. One day when it blew up, it formed like a black smoke, a big, black cloud, and a lot of people had respiratory problems.

That's when I started noticing that I couldn't hold my bladder. And this kept on happening, kept on happening, while we was over there. Then when we got back to the States, my soldiers started complaining, and they was sent to the hospital, sent to psych, told it was all in their head.

I kept on dealing with it, and one day it really hurt me and struck me. I was coming from fishing with my son, and I wasn't even a block away from the Seven-Eleven in San Antonio, Texas, and I couldn't even make it to the Seven-Eleven, and I soiled on myself. Then I knew then there was something terrible wrong with me.

Then as I went on with my bowel and bladder problem, I realized what was going on, and when I ran into some of the individuals that was in my unit, some of the guys, I would pull them aside and ask them if they was having some of the same problems. I said, "You can tell me if you want to, you know, but you don't have to tell me." And all of them that I spoke to said yes, they was having the same problems and some more problems. And I told them, I said, "Well, you need to get rid of your pride and go forward and tell people, go tell the doctor about what's going on because you and I is not the only one."

I went to have a rectal exam, and they found nerve damage to my internal sphincter muscle. The sphincter muscle is the one that helps hold your bowel. So when you have to go to the bathroom or get the urge to go, you have to be whupped in the bathroom, or you'd best be running, or you just go on yourself. And I know that a forty-four-year-old, I'm forty-four years old now, and I know there's forty-four-year-old men that haven't been to the Gulf War don't have this problem. It started when I came back, and I know it happened over there because there's too many of us having the same problem. And I have to buy expensive diapers and stuff. The government's not buying diapers for me.

I miss a lot of events with my kids, you know, their activities. My son plays college football. Could you imagine me going to a college football game, eighty, ninety thousand people trying to get into the same restroom with you? No, I'd soil on myself. So all of these activities and things that my kids have been into since I've been back and the things that I've missed, no one can give that back to me, no one.

I got to where I couldn't even hardly breathe, I would get like caught up or choked, like my breath was cut off. It's just so much, you know, my migraines, my rash, my poor circulation. My legs swell up for no reason. I had two surgeons from Walter Reed come down, and they tell me, "Sergeant Twymon, we don't know what's going on." And I said, "Well, you the doctors, I don't know what's going on either."

I had a bone marrow test. My platelets was turning over so fast, and the blood specialist didn't know why. I got anemic and had a liver biopsy.

I was very healthy prior to going over there. I used to run everyday. I used to lift weights, like I had a weight machine in my garage. Since I've been back, they have had to go into my knees due to joint problems where my cartilage has been ate all up for some reason. I have a hole in my median condial for an unknown reason. My bone's deteriorating, and my teeth are rotting from the inside out.

I always have tried to be faithful to my country, just like President Kennedy, whom I admired, he always said, "Ask not what your country can do for you, what you can do for your country." Well, that's the way I grew up, I was brought up. And, sad to say, I went and did for my country, but my country's not doing for me. They don't care. They don't care. We just a number. I guess the soonest we can die, they'll be better off, you know, the government, because there's so many of us. And I'm tired of them trying to hide everything because the proof is there, you look at all the soldiers that have been over there and are sick. And the sad thing about it is, you get back here and you're sick and you go to get some more insurance policy, and you can't even get insurance because of your illness or because you was in Desert Storm. And that's sad. What can a person leave back for their family to continue on to live the life that they was living if they can't get insurance?

Since I've been back from the Gulf War, I also notice that lots of things bother me that never bothered me before. Different perfume, different cologne, gas, different smell of even smoke or cigarettes, I just automatically get sick, and sometime it takes me days or weeks to recover.

One day I was on an elevator, and someone got on there with some loud perfume. Then all of a sudden it hit me. I got lightheaded and I was breathing difficult, so I went to my office to sit down. And then I was still feeling lightheaded, so I went outside to see if I could get some air so I'd be all right. Then when I came back, I was still lightheaded, so I went over to ASU, which is right around the hall from the operating room. And the nurses over there took my blood pressure. They didn't say nothing at first, just put my feet up. Then they took it again. Then next thing I knew, one was on the phone, and here come a wheelchair, and they was rolling me down to the emergency room because they thought I was having a heart attack. They started putting IVs in me, putting EKGs on me, nitro, nitroglycerin. And I was in the hospital for about four or five days for that, and that wasn't the first time that had happened, with the chest pain, reaction and all that.

It's like, it's rough. A lot of people don't understand it, but it's real, and it's not in my head neither. And that's what I think a lot of people need to understand. We're not making this up. There's too many of us. I don't know what the government is going to do, but I hope they hurry up and do something soon because there's too many of us that have served our country proudly, and now we're living like we're third-class citizens.

Sue

Medical Transcriptionist

When Alison Johnson asked if I would like to write my MCS story for this book, I initially hesitated to do so because I was concerned that my story might discourage some chemically sensitive people and diminish their hope for a full recovery. But after a long internal debate, I felt a strong need to tell the truth about this insidious and horrific illness that destroys lives at every level: financially, socially, emotionally, and most of all physically. I wanted to come out of hiding in hopes of helping others struggling with this "hidden epidemic."

Too many people with MCS live on the fringes of society, and the people we encounter often treat us as if our chemical sensitivity is a sign of mental instability. Some of us are better able to cope with MCS than others, depending on the financial or emotional support we receive, but this illness continuously forces one to seek all the depths of inner strength one can muster. For me, there have been days when finding that strength has been impossible. I have found very little support from the medical community other than alternative practitioners. After struggling for fourteen years, the exhaustion of the challenge sometimes becomes unbearable to me. I realize not everyone who is suffering from serious chemical sensitivity feels this way, but I know from experience that I am not alone. Others not fearful of being honest have shared their stories with me.

My MCS story starts in 1994 in San Diego, California. I would characterize myself at that time in my life as an intelligent, outgoing female extremely conscious of fashion, devoted to family and friends, with a need to please others. My husband, Norm, who is also outgoing, is a very big part of my story. He suffers from chronic fatigue syndrome and a mild form of MCS. Where exactly our exposure began is elusive. Physicians we have consulted have mentioned various reasons for our chronic ill health: 1) We lived on a golf course for nine years, so this heavy exposure to pesticides is the most likely source of our health problems. 2) My husband and I may have both been exposed to a virus that compromised our immune systems. 3) My husband's exposure to Agent Orange in Vietnam might be a factor.

In 1994, Norm was diagnosed with mononucleosis; he was later diagnosed with chronic mono and then given the diagnosis of chronic fatigue syndrome. He was completely bedridden for the first year after he contracted mono. Within six months of the time he became ill, I also became ill and incapacitated with similar symptoms, but a physician immediately diagnosed me with MCS.

In a matter of months, Norm and I went from living the American dream to almost being homeless. With both of us sick, we had no income and lost everything. Norm was unable to collect disability from his private insurance because the diagnosis of chronic fatigue syndrome was considered controversial. Appeals to the insurance company and letters to politicians fell on deaf ears. I was able to collect workers' compensation for a short period of time, and that enabled us to buy groceries, but I was expected to go back to work as soon as possible.

My symptoms were so debilitating and bizarre that it was difficult for friends and family to understand my condition. The fatigue and weakness were so overwhelming that I could barely walk. I had intense burning in my eyes, inside my nose, and in my upper respiratory tract; it felt as if I were suffering from chemical burns. For almost a year, I suffered from daily fevers, chills, and a cough. My burden was increased by my struggle with the health-care bureaucracy and misdiagnoses and misunderstandings. Dealing with health-care providers who had little understanding of chemical sensitivity was frustrating and often humiliating.

Having been refused help of any kind and having no financial resources, we continued to try to work while we were sick. Since I had worked as a medical transcriptionist in the past, I decided to try performing this work at home so that I could avoid the chemical exposures I would encounter in a office setting. Workers' comp agreed to purchase new equipment for me to use in my home, but little did I realize what would happen next. Within a few minutes of turning on the new computer and printer, I almost passed out from the strong plastic odors given off by the new equipment. My knees buckled, and I had immediate diarrhea. I soon realized that I could not be near the equipment without experiencing serious symptoms, but in desperation I tried to make the situation work and continued to use the computer and printer for eight hours a day during the next year. The more I sat in front of the computer, however, the more intense my eye pain became. I was repeatedly diagnosed with allergic conjunctivitis and was treated with steroid eye drops to no avail. I developed allergies to all the other eye drops my doctor prescribed.

It was clear at this point that I couldn't keep working from my home. Since neither Norm nor I was able to get approval from Social Security disability or private disability because of the controversy surrounding MCS and CFS, we decided we had no choice but to return to Maine, where we had grown up. We returned to Maine with no money and no belongings and were taken in by relatives. Our eighteen-year-old daughter made the decision to stay in California completely alone, and the stress of that on me was excruciating. Also, our son was going through a painful divorce at that time. Our tight-bonded family was falling apart at the seams. Explaining our illness to our children and extended family was challenging. Although they tried to be supportive, they were unable to fathom this alien illness. How could we expect others to comprehend this emerging illness when we could not? How could they understand when we did not?

By now, I could no longer sleep in a bed or on a couch without experiencing symptoms of dizziness, nausea, twitching, headache, and brain fog because when I lay down, my nose was right next to synthetic mattresses or cushions. I was reduced to sleeping on the floor, which was of course not very comfortable.

There were times when I wanted to set up a tent on a mountain top because all I could tolerate was fresh air. My life seemed like a living hell at this point. Socializing with others means a tremendous amount to me, but now my social contacts had to be sharply reduced because I could no longer tolerate the perfume and other scented products most people use. It would be a long time before I could educate myself of MCS and understand what I needed to do to take care of myself. My husband was in complete denial of his own illness and was mainly concerned about working and taking care of financial matters.

When we returned to Maine, we vigorously pursued the goal of trying to get back to work, even when it meant ignoring our symptoms. We both lied to employers in order to get work, and we tried to present a happy and normal façade in order to fool everyone. I found a job working as a medical transcriptionist in a hospital. Being in sales, my husband was able to come home during the day and take frequent naps, but he was literally dragging himself to and from work. I worked at the local hospital even though I was sick and in pain everyday. Our years of acting in community theater now provided us with the ability to play act our way through daily life, or so we thought.

After living with relatives for six months, we finally moved into our own apartment. For furniture, we could afford only a sofa and a mattress, and we had to use a cardboard box for our living room table.

We had reconciled ourselves to our losses, and we were just happy to have each other. We thought this would be our new start, but that was not to be. My first night in that apartment was like the *Titanic*'s maiden voyage. The new paint, carpet cleaners, and other chemical fumes made me deathly ill. Unfortunately, I still had not learned what kind of chemical exposures I should be avoiding and had chosen an apartment too quickly because I was so eager to get back to "normal," living in our own place.

I moved out of the apartment immediately but had nowhere to go. Friends and relatives could not understand what was happening to me and were sure I was having a nervous breakdown. The eye pain I had been experiencing for three years became so intense that thoughts of death were becoming more frequent. I was reduced to living with various relatives and once again became homeless. I had nowhere to turn. My husband was trying to do everything he could to help me, but to no avail. Going from one doctor to another was useless. Traditional medicine found little clinical evidence that I was sick. Doctors would roll their eyes and not look directly at me while saying, "I cannot find anything physically wrong with you."

I started feeling extremely hopeless and was convinced I was a complete burden to my husband and family. My attempt to return to a normal life was failing, and I had nowhere to turn. To make matters worse, I went to work one day and found that the hospital had just installed twelve new computers in the room where I worked. The outgassing fumes were so strong that I could only work for a couple of hours before I had to leave. It was clear that I could no longer keep up the façade. I could barely walk and knew I could never return to that office. As I shuffled out of the office, hopelessness, despair, and loneliness took center stage in my life. I could not bear the thought of any more losses. It seemed as if everything that had brought me joy would never again return. No more makeup, no more hair dye, no nail polish, no hairspray, no synthetic clothing, no more dancing in clubs, no more cocktail parties, no more high fashion, no more family gatherings. Most difficult to deal with was the embarrassment of having to try and explain to friends and family what was happening when I could see that no one believed me.

Having run out of options to normalize my life, I started planning my suicide before I left the hospital where I had worked. I thought this would solve all of my problems and I would no longer be a burden to anyone ever again. Most important of all, I would no longer have to endure the unbearable eye pain. It would all be over soon. I planned what I thought would be the perfect suicide with an overdose of pills away from home. I felt an incredible sense of relief and comfort knowing my struggle was almost over.

I asked a friend in an apartment down the hall if I could sleep over there while she was away for the weekend. I did feel a bit better in her apartment so that's the excuse I gave my husband. About 9 P.M., I went into her apartment and swallowed sixty pills–painkillers and sleeping pills. I put suicide notes to my husband and children on the coffee table, lay down on the couch, arms on my chest, pillow under my head, and fell into a blissful, effortless sleep. To my dismay, I woke up a few days later in an intensive care unit and realized that Norm had found me in time to save my life. The following is a copy of the note I had left for him:

To My Precious Husband,

I had planned to write you a long letter but that is useless at this time. One thing you and I never had a problem with was talking. In these last few days, there isn't anything that hasn't been talked about other than my actual death.

As I've told you, I love you more than life itself. You have been my best best best friend for almost 30 years, the person I have depended on for everything (and you have always delivered the goods), my adviser, my confessor, my therapist, MY EVERYTHING.

There are no more words to be said. I will not put them down on paper as they are OUR precious and private moments together that I will never share with anyone else.

[*Editor's note: I have not included a list that appeared here containing specific instructions about matters like cremation.*]

Whatever will be, will be. I won't be the first person to have tried this nor the last. I only wish I had had someone to help me so that it would be a sure thing without any pain or suffering. I always kidded about Jack Kevorkian but I sure wish I had him on my side but, unfortunately, I don't. I only have you and I would never have involved you in my decision. This was my decision and my decision alone.

I am fed up with being a burden to you, a burden to my children, useless in society. I have loved life too much and have lived life too fully to live like this, a pitiful existence from day to day, not knowing what depressing thing the next day will bring, not knowing when I can no longer work, not knowing if we are going to lose our apartment because of not working after we have already lost everything there is to lose.

I worship you and thank you for standing behind me and being the support system that you were. However, there comes a time when enough is enough. I now bring only negative to everyone's lives and can no longer tolerate doing that. If I cannot live a quality and productive life then there is no life left for me.

I kiss the ground you walk on. I will be with you always and I pray to God that I will not be punished for what I have done and that we can someday be reunited in our love again. You have been the most wonderful thing that has happened to me in my life. I thank God that he gave you to me for 30 years. A more perfect husband never existed. You have been a perfect husband, perfect provider and perfect father.

If I fail at my suicide attempt, I beg you to please continue to love me until I finally succeed. I could not bear to be in the hospital alone. I love you.

                                                    Sue

After I had recovered physically, I was transferred to a psychiatric facility, as state law requires. In my opinion, I received little or no help from the doctors or staff there. It was merely a warehouse where one was held until such time that they heard the words they wanted to hear, such as "I regret what I did" or "I won't do it again." I quickly learned to play their game and was discharged before long. After my discharge, Norm told me what happened "that" night.

Norm had gone to bed in our apartment down the hall from my friend's apartment where I was sleeping. He sensed something was not quite right, but tried to sleep anyway. At 3 A.M., according to the clock, he bolted out of bed, got up, and rushed to the apartment I was in without knowing why. He turned the doorknob and realized I had not locked it. When he walked into the kitchen, he saw the empty prescription bottles. He ran to the couch and found me lying there, breathing in a shallow and erratic way with saliva on both sides of my mouth. He at once called 9-1-1. A locked door might have ended my story here.

It took that experience to awaken me to the fact that I could no longer keep working and to realize that suicide was not the solution to that problem. I was determined to learn about disability income possibilities, and I decided to contact other MCS individuals who had succeeded in attaining such disability income. I wrote a short description of my case and sent it to a physician in California who, along with an attorney in Florida, agreed to help me obtain Social Security disability income. Both women did this for me free of charge, and I will forever be indebted to them.

This is when things finally started turning around. I now had the time to educate myself and to start seeing alternative physicians and learn how to deal with all the challenges I was faced with. I managed to make many changes in my life and slowly started feeling much better. I was not back to normal by any stretch of the imagination, but was able to start functioning in the "modern world" once again as long as I had my safe haven with limited chemical exposures to come home to. Socializing has always been of the utmost importance to me, so spending time with friends and family was a priority. It was difficult, however, to balance my desire and need to spend time with others with my need to limit chemical exposures. I experienced good days, bad days, good months, bad months, periods of healing after daring to be out and about in our toxic world.

In the meantime, Norm was becoming sicker and sicker, experiencing a downward spiral with alcohol abuse. Denial worked for a while until he too broke down emotionally and physically. Luckily, he had a physician who understood chronic fatigue syndrome and helped him obtain disability income within a few months. Needless to say, however, two Social Security disability incomes do not go very far and did not enable us to spend the money required to minimize our chemical exposures in our living quarters.

After searching for a year, we did find an older apartment that had not been renovated or recently painted and appeared to be relatively safe. It was our dream come true. For the next four years, life was the best it had been in a long time. It definitely was not without its challenges, but I was able to work through them. My depression lifted, and I was able to volunteer as a buyer in a hospital gift shop and travel to various states on buying trips. My husband learned how to deal with his illness and cherished his life of sobriety. However, it was all a daily juggling act. Living in isolation was not an option that either one of us wanted. We learned to accept our limitations and losses and worked around them.

By the fifth year, the unexpected happened. (Never get too comfortable with MCS; it is always lurking in the wings.) Our landlord decided to renovate the exterior of the building with vinyl siding. I kept telling myself that everything would be OK, but that was not the case.

Within two days of the new insulation and new siding being applied, I became very ill. Once again I felt like I was going to pass out all the time and experienced extreme weakness and lethargy. I also started having gastrointestinal symptoms, difficulty eating many foods, and problems being around plastic products. I had been designing and making beaded jewelry, but suddenly found that I could no longer even touch the beads without getting symptoms. I was reacting to everything in my environment and once again found myself homeless. I started sleeping at my mother's house, and we even stayed in a motel for short periods. Five months later, with the onset of winter, which meant that the vinyl siding was outgassing less, I was able to return to the apartment with less severe symptoms. I was never really able, however, to regain my health. Once again we started searching for another apartment but had little success. Most apartments offered for rent have recently been painted or remodeled, and there were many other potential hazards in the various apartments we looked at. Renting a home was out of the question due to our limited funds.

Then one day I thought luck had come our way when I found what I thought was going to be the perfect apartment. It was older and charming, and it contained no carpeting and had not been recently painted. It was more then we could afford, but I was willing to sacrifice in other areas in order to have a safe home. What little money we had left was used for moving. Unfortunately, my luck was short-lived. Within two days of moving into the apartment, I became deathly ill once again. We later found out that the apartment was full of mold, but I was unaware of this when we moved in.

Since I could barely walk and felt like I had perpetual flu symptoms, I had to leave the apartment during the day and sleep at my mother's home at night. Norm was so discouraged. He had worked his fingers to the bone moving us in, we had spent our last dollar on this apartment, and now I was totally discouraged and in a state of depression. Again, the embarrassment of trying to explain all this to family members was too much to bear. Nobody knew what to say or do with me. I was homeless and totally hopeless. I felt like I could no longer continue this vicious cycle. Once again I decided that I couldn't bear being a burden to Norm and my family, so I planned to take an overdose of pills and this time do it where absolutely no one would find me. My two suicide attempts were not cries for help. Both were planned so that no one would find me in time to thwart my intentions, but Norm found me both times. The following is a copy of my last suicide note:

Dear Norm, Parrish, and Gabrielle,

If you are reading this note, the first thing I ask is for your forgiveness, in fact, I beg you. The three of you are the light of my life but I cannot bear to be a further burden to the three of you and especially to Dad.

    I don't think that you know exactly what my life has dwindled down to except for Dad. I have been getting progressively worse since January, and I'm at the point where I can't even be living in a house. I am reacting to everything in the universe. My stomach, intestines, diaphragm and rib cages constantly swell on a daily basis causing a lot of pain and difficulty breathing. I cannot sit on furniture anymore other than a wooden chair because I react to foam and rubber. I cannot make my jewelry anymore because I react to the plastic containers and plastic beads. I react to the plastic when playing Scrabble. I cannot use my cell phone or go to the movies or near a TV–especially I cannot drive without experiencing pain due to the electromagnetic fields. I am worse in this apartment in terms of pain in my rib cage. My life has been reduced to sitting in a wooden chair and reading a book. I am now reacting to my clothes and have nothing to wear that doesn't bother me. I can't keep moving from house to house.

    I refuse to go live out in the desert, sleeping in a tent as my counterparts do and sleeping in a car.

    Dad has been an absolute pillar for me lately. He takes on burden after burden without complaint so that I can get well but to no avail. I pray to God that I will be reconnected with him in another life. I pray that I am reconnected with you Parrish and Gabrielle. The emotional pain that I am experiencing is indescribable.

    I love you all so much, but I guess I'm too weak to keep going. I've done it for 12 years and I've given it my best but I can't do it anymore. This illness has totally broken me and again I ask for your forgiveness for my weakness.

    Please take care of Dad and each other with lots of love and closeness. That is all I ask. I am 100% totally responsible for this action. I am exhausted at trying to keep up appearances of being normal. I was successful at it for a long time but I cannot do it for one more day. Please tell my family I love them.

I adore you Gabrielle
I adore you Parrish
Most of all, I idolize you Norm. You have been my
EVERYTHING.
   Please promise me to love each other dearly.

                              Love,
                              Mom

Norm later told me the details about that nightmarish day when I tried
once again to take my life. When he had come home from his part-time
job at about 4 P.M., the apartment was empty. An eerie feeling
immediately settled over him. He had stopped by earlier in the day and
had found me despondent and a bit detached. He had gone back to work
with my words circling in his head all day: "Its my problem, and I will
take care of it." Within ten minutes after coming home from work, he
checked the medicine cabinet and knew at once what had happened. He
called 9-1-1 immediately. A picture of me and a car description were
given to the police, and they found my car in a local motel parking lot.
The paramedics told Norm that in another half hour it would have been
too late.
   After my discharge from the intensive care unit, I was once again
transferred to a psychiatric facility, this time one located in a town thirty
miles away. My experience there was much more enlightening then the
one in the psychiatric facility where I was placed after my first suicide
attempt. The physicians and staff seemed to understand MCS and
actually discussed my symptoms and tried to do some problem solving
along with me. The psychiatrist sat down with Norm and me and
explained that my condition was called "situational depression." He
explained that when my physical symptoms are kept at bay, I am pretty
much my old self–happy and contented–and can go on with my daily
living, but when my MCS symptoms become acute, I immediately fall
into this abyss where I feel like I've reached the point of no return.
   While I was in the hospital, Norm had tested our apartment with
mold Petri dishes, and the results showed eight different mold species.
He confronted the landlord, who dissolved our lease immediately with
no argument.
   What do you do after two failed suicide attempts? Antidepressants
have never been an option because they make me extremely ill. The
only thing I could do was to change my mindset. I had to search within
myself deeper then I had ever searched. I had to find strength that I did

not know existed. I had no choice but to face my challenges head on. Once again I moved in with relatives, and I also visited Arizona on a number of occasions. I have considered moving there, but there are as many positives and negatives in that region as there are in Maine. There is no perfect place for the chemically sensitive. Recently, with a great deal of research and creativity, my husband and I were able to qualify for a low-income mortgage loan, and we found a small older home that we could purchase. The home has not been without its challenges, but we do have more control over our safety then we did in an apartment. I do not know how long we will be able to afford to stay there, but for the time being it is workable.

My journey has taken me from living the good life on a golf course in sunny California to an old, outdated house built in 1959. I have learned to lower my expectations about everything in life and feel that I am a better person for it. I am just thankful to have a roof over my head and food on the table and to enjoy a simple movie or planting flowers. Fourteen years later, I still cannot sleep in a bed, but I am thankful for my cot. I know that my gypsy lifestyle is far from over and that my safe haven is temporary. Who knows where the future will take me? When I feel sad, I think of those who are so sick that they must live outside or in their cars and then I realize how fortunate I am. I am more hopeful at this point and more willing to let go and accept what may come my way. Most of all, I am so appreciative for the one constant in my life–my husband, who has supported me 100 percent and never stops trying to make things work for me. Although he is on disability, he works part-time so that we can continue to live in a relatively safe environment. None of this would be possible without him. I sometimes think how difficult my life would be without him, but I try not to linger on such thoughts. I hope if that day ever presents itself that my survivor instinct will kick in. But for now, I live by the AA motto, "One day at a time."

Norm's account: As I write this, we are about to celebrate forty-one years of marriage. I am still naïve enough to believe that our relationship is what movies and poems are about. Many self-help books are written about being married, but Sue and I are the epilogues to all those books.

After forty-one years, I still have the same burning commitment to make Sue happy because she deserves it. Her qualities and values throughout and in spite of this illness radiate at the most difficult times. Her empathy and love for others, her honest and supportive relationship with those around her is unfaltering, whether it be friends or family. Their needs are her needs. Recently, her eighty-three-year-old mother was quite ill, and in spite of Sue's own illness, she was at the hospital every day even though the hospital disinfectants made her sicker. To love Sue is a gift.

The "give and take" of a relationship has taken on a new meaning for me. In the first thirty years of our marriage, my instincts were to "give" a home, security, vacations, love, etc. All of these are found in marital handbooks.

After MCS came into our lives some fifteen years ago, I learned about "taking." I try to take away her pain, her despair, her loneliness, and most important of all I want to take away her feeling that she is a burden. Having a mild form of MCS myself, I have never doubted her symptoms, and I know how real they are.

Yes, Sue's two attempted suicides were the most heart-wrenching and painful experiences I have ever lived through, but after the second attempt I have a new mission. Like Sue, I also had to change my thinking and search myself for inner strength. Since her diagnosis of "situational depression," my mission is to "take away" that "situation" before it becomes overwhelming. To quote from the book of poetry titled *The Prophet*, which was written by Sue's and my favorite author, Kahlil Gibran:

To know the pain of too much tenderness
To be wounded by your own understanding of love
And to bleed willingly and joyfully
To wake at dawn with a winged heart and give thanks
    for another day of living
To return home at eventide and gratitude
And then to sleep with a prayer for the beloved in your heart and a song
    of praise upon your lips.

Lindsay Huckabee

FEMA Trailer Exposure

The first part of Lindsay Huckabee's story consists of her July 19, 2007, testimony to the Government Reform and Oversight Committee of the U.S. House of Representatives.

I would like to start by thanking Chairman Waxman and the members of the committee for taking the time to address this issue and for allowing me the honor of coming before you to speak. My name is Lindsay Huckabee. I live in Kiln, Mississippi in a single-wide mobile home provided by the Federal Emergency Management Agency (FEMA) following Hurricane Katrina with my husband and our five children.

On August 29, 2005, I lived in an apartment in Pass Christian, Mississippi. A few days later, we learned that our apartment and all of its contents were destroyed by Hurricane Katrina. The floodwaters had come into our apartment and above the ceiling several feet into the apartment above ours. We contacted FEMA and were granted immediate assistance. In early October, we received a travel trailer to use as our temporary residence. Because of the many maintenance problems the trailer had, we were unable to stay in it. After six weeks of no response from the maintenance department, we contacted FEMA. We were told that we qualified for a single-wide mobile home because of our family size. If we cleared a site, provided our own septic, water and power to the site, they would deliver a home. We met all of the requirements and were ready for the trailer by mid-November.

On December 14, 2005, our new home was delivered and set up. We were very excited and felt very blessed. We had four children and another due at the end of February. As we were moving into the trailer, we noticed that it had a very strong odor. We figured that is what a "new" trailer smelled like. Our whole family began to have sinus problems, our eyes would burn and water, and our throats were constantly sore. We seemed to catch every cold and virus going around, but we couldn't get rid of the illnesses. Three of our children began having

severe nosebleeds, sometimes three or four times a week. I began having
migraine headaches and pre-term labor. At the time, my doctor thought
maybe my blood pressure was going up at home, causing the headaches.

After three weeks of pre-term labor stopped by medication, my
youngest son Michael was delivered four weeks early on January 17,
2006. Each of my previous pregnancies was either full term or past due.
Michael was healthy and came home on time. Within a few days of
being home, his sinuses were congested. I was so scared. None of my
children even had a cold until they were much older than he was at the
time. I kept thinking he is so small and too young to be so sick. He never
had a fever though, which suggested that his sinuses were just irritated.
I was so worried that he would choke on the phlegm he was coughing
up that I stayed up most nights watching him sleep.

My daughter Lelah, who was four when we received the trailer,
seemed to be affected the most. She began having asthma symptoms.
She had been diagnosed with asthma when she was about one, but had
been symptom free for about a year. Just prior to moving into the mobile
home, I discussed with her doctor the possibility that she had outgrown
the asthma when we went in to see him for her four-year-old checkup.
Over the next 18 months, Lelah had more ear infections than I can
count, nosebleeds several times a month, sometimes as many as a three
a week. She had pneumonia several times. For most of the cases, she
was treated at home with steroids and breathing treatments, but she had
to be hospitalized twice because the pneumonia was so severe. Lelah
was sent to an ENT [Ear, Nose, Throat physician], where she underwent
allergy testing, an MRI, and surgery to put tubes in her ears so that the
excess fluid her sinuses were producing had a place to escape. She was
put on different allergy medications, steroids, and nasal sprays to try
and ease her symptoms. Nothing worked. I was told by our ENT that we
needed to get out of the trailer as soon as we could. He had many repeat
patients with the same symptoms all living in FEMA trailers. He said
that there were chemicals that could be making Lelah sick. We took
Lelah to an allergy and asthma specialist. He did another allergy test and
found nothing. I never thought I would be upset to hear that nothing was
wrong with my child after a test. If there were an allergy, then at least
we would know what to fight. He did say that her asthma was not as
under control as I thought it was. Her coughing in the middle of the
night and the constant "cold" she kept needed to be closely monitored.

He said that she obviously had a constant exposure to some sort of irritant. Then he asked if we were in a FEMA trailer. He too had seen an increase of patients with inactive or mild asthma having more severe problems upon moving into these trailers. After putting Lelah on inhaled steroids twice a day, a daily allergy medication, and an oral steroid if she starts to get a cold, we have her asthma "under control." Lelah missed 42 days of kindergarten this year. All but three of these were because of doctor visits or asthma systems. The school nurse called me to get her from school several times because of nosebleeds and fevers. Looking back, she would have been better off spending more time at school rather than being sent home. We were taking a sick child and making her spend more time in the place that made her sick.

After months and months of office visits and phone calls, I was frustrated and upset. I came home one afternoon to find my daughter covering her nose; her hands, arms and shirt were covered in blood. The surprising part is that I did not feel the need to rush to her and find out what was wrong. I did not think for a second that it was anything more than a bloody nose. Two years ago, I would have panicked trying to get to her. Later that night, I cried for hours. How had we gotten to the point where I was not surprised to see my child covered in blood? I asked my doctor what I was doing wrong. Why couldn't I get my kids healthy and keep them that way? I had always been one of those moms who wouldn't bother the doctor with a low-grade fever or a cold that didn't last more than a week. Before moving into the FEMA trailer, I can't remember going to the doctor other than for well-child checks and a few times with Lelah when she was very young for treatment of her asthma. Suddenly I was at the doctor's office or calling him just about every week. The receptionist knew me by my first name, and I swear she probably knew my voice, too. Our pediatric doctor had told me that there seemed to be a trend among patients in FEMA trailers and increased office visits with allergy-like symptoms. It was through him that a Sierra Club member contacted me about a formaldehyde test to see if we were living in levels that could be dangerous. I really did not want this to be the answer, since we had nowhere else to go.

We finally had a formaldehyde test done on our trailer in April of 2007. It came back as 0.18ppm—well above the 0.10ppm believed to be harmful to humans. There is no way to know how high it was in the 16 months we lived in the trailer. Since FEMA suggested that "opening windows would out-gas the fumes and lower the level," I have to believe that the level was much higher when we moved in. When we told FEMA about the test, we met much opposition. FEMA representatives were rude when I called them. I was forced to call more than 5 different representatives, and my request for a new mobile home was lost twice before anything was done to help solve my problem. Finally, FEMA agreed to replace our mobile home. We packed up our stuff and put it in storage. We stayed with family for the week it took to switch the trailers out. We were told that the new trailer would be "formaldehyde free." It was a used trailer built in 2005 by a different company. We had a formaldehyde test done on it before we started to move anything into it. An inspector from FEMA saw the tester hanging and asked what it was. When I told him it was used to test for formaldehyde, he said that people were claiming to have high formaldehyde levels so they could get bigger and better trailers. When I asked if FEMA had done tests to find this out, he said no. The test on the new trailer came back at 0.108ppm which is still above the level believed to be harmful, but lower than the last trailer. When we called FEMA to tell them what the results were, the lady said, "so we are good, right?'

Three weeks ago my husband was having his teeth cleaned when the dentist found a mass in his soft palette. He was referred to an ENT to have it examined. He had a CT scan followed by surgery to remove the mass, which they discovered was a polymorphic adenoma tumor. My husband is a healthy, 30-year-old nonsmoker. His tumor was a common type, but in a very rare location. When I brought up our recent formaldehyde test, the ENT asked my husband if he breathes through his mouth which he sometimes does. While no one can say for certain that the formaldehyde caused this kind of mouth tumor, the ENT said that he will definitely make note of it for possible future study. It is known, however, that formaldehyde puts people at an increased risk for nasal and lung cancer. Mouth tumors could be another long-term effect of people living with the high concentrations of formaldehyde.

What makes me so angry is that FEMA is providing trailers to disaster victims that they have "inspected" and deemed safe without truly ensuring that they are. FEMA does not run air quality tests on the homes they provide; my air quality test was done at the expense of the Sierra Club. I have heard there is a pamphlet that was given to people by FEMA about formaldehyde, but I never received one, not even with the second trailer. If it had not been for my family's medical problems, I would not have known about the formaldehyde problem. I am scared to think of how many other families are being exposed to high levels of formaldehyde and will have medical problems in the future.

What scares me even more is the knowledge that the level of 0.1ppm, the maximum recommended exposure limit, was not intended to gauge how safe exposure was for children, people with breathing problems, or even healthy adults for longer than the average eight hour workday. No one can tell us what to expect long-term from this exposure. I do not want to believe that FEMA knew about the formaldehyde when they issued these homes, but I do know that when it was brought to their attention, they spent little effort to fix the problem. Instead, people were made to feel that they were being too picky, or looking to blame someone else for simple colds and normal problems. When FEMA took on the role of landlord for the thousands of people, they took on the responsibility to provide a safe, fit home for these people. This temporary housing should have given people time to get on their feet again, and even save some money for a permanent home. Instead we are spending so much on medical bills and prescriptions, we are actually moving backwards.

Thank you very much for taking the time to read my testimony and to deal with this very important issue.

Lindsay's April 1, 2008, testimony to the House Committee on Science and Technology, included these passages that shed additional light on the family's health:

My daughter Vicki is 13 years old and has had a sore throat off and on since moving into the first FEMA trailer. Vicki keeps mild congestion in her sinuses and has been on antibiotics several times, but has never been hospitalized.

My daughter Caitlin will be nine this month, she has had sinus infections, pneumonia, asthmatic bronchitis, sore throat, nose bleeds, headaches and asthmatic symptoms. Caitlin is currently on a daily allergy medication and inhaled asthma medication as needed. Prior to living in the trailers Caitlin had never been treated for any breathing problems. Caitlin has had many x-rays and been on antibiotics again and again, but she has only been hospitalized once.

Lelah is six years old and since moving in to our first FEMA trailer she has developed moderate asthma and has also had sinus infections severe enough to need an operation to widen her sinus passages. Lelah's doctor said that with the sinus tissue staying inflamed from the constant irritation, there was nowhere for the sinus fluid to drain. Lelah has had pneumonia, ear infections, throat infections, asthmatic bronchitis, nose bleeds, headaches, two MRIs and has been put under for surgery four times. Lelah is currently on three daily medications with two more as needed. In the past Lelah has been on as many as eight daily medications at one time and she has been hospitalized three times.

Steven is four years old and has been pretty fortunate health wise. Steven is on a daily allergy medication and he has had asthmatic bronchitis, pneumonia, sinus infections and nose bleeds. Steven has also been treated with breathing treatments for asthma. Prior to living in the FEMA trailers Steven had never had breathing problems of any kind. Steven has only been hospitalized once.

Michael is two years old and he was born prematurely after we moved into our FEMA trailer. Michael has had sinus infections off and on since he was six days old; he has also had asthmatic bronchitis, pneumonia, laryngitis, only a few nosebleeds and undergone cardiac testing because he occasionally turns blue for an unknown reason. Michael is currently on two daily allergy medications, a nasal steroid, and antibiotics for the sixth straight week. Michael has been hospitalized three times.

After returning from Washington, D.C., in July of 2007, we received information from FEMA on formaldehyde. The information sheet gave a number for FEMA to call for more details on what levels were acceptable and what the long-term health effects would be. The number proved to be useless. After talking to the woman at FEMA about our symptoms and our concerns we were told that it did not sound like we had a problem with formaldehyde. We had already had a test done on our trailer so we knew what our problem was. We were told that we did not qualify for the formaldehyde-testing program. We then asked what level was considered safe for us to live in and her response was "I don't know; you have to call the CDC for that information." We called the CDC number we were given and it proved to be as useless as the FEMA number. First we were told to call FEMA. After insisting that we had already called them and been told to call the CDC number, we were transferred to six different desks of people in different departments and levels of management where the final answer we received was that we needed to talk to FEMA about our concerns. The CDC representatives said that they did not have information on levels of formaldehyde and what was safe and what was not. We were told that the employees could not give us their names or even an employee number. Therefore there was no way for us to follow up on the conversations or have anyone to hold accountable for the lack of information.

I was able to meet with several CDC officers at a meeting held in Bay St. Louis, Mississippi on March 6, 2008. I found them very willing to answer our questions about the formaldehyde and possible effects on people. I was surprised to learn how little is known about formaldehyde and long-term effects. While searching for the magic "safe" level of formaldehyde, we found several different numbers through the internet. The level of 0.1ppm, the most commonly accepted safe limit, was not intended to gauge how safe exposure was for children, people with breathing problems, or even healthy adults for longer than the average workday. According to the CDC representative I spoke with at the community meeting that was held to answer questions about formaldehyde, there is "no safe level for exposure in a residence." I was told at the meeting that CDC was not aware of the issue until after the July 17 hearing last year. I personally find this hard to believe. It is my understanding that the ATSDR [Agency for Toxic Substances and Disease Registry] did the original testing for FEMA and OSHA when they wanted to know what the levels were for employees and how to bring them down. They reported the levels to FEMA and agreed to not share the information. They even sent a revised letter making sure the FEMA knew that there was no known SAFE level for people to live in since formaldehyde is a known carcinogen. ATSDR is a part of CDC. According to everything I can find on the CDC and ATSDR, both claim to exist to protect us from toxic substances—like formaldehyde. What I can't understand is, how an agency set in place to protect the people, failed to let the people know about this problem. I did not think it was there to help the government find out how much it messed up and then help them keep quiet about it. I know that at least one pediatrician contacted the CDC to find out about starting a study and researching what was going on down here with the kids in the FEMA travel trailers and mobile homes.

There is now evidence that FEMA knew about the formaldehyde as early as December of 2005, which is the same time that I got my first mobile home. They covered up the problem, hid behind lawyers and made sure they could not be held responsible. FEMA made people feel like they were being picky, and ungrateful for mentioning the illnesses and requesting assistance. While FEMA was covering their behinds, my children were staying sick. I blamed myself for not doing enough to keep them well, but when FEMA took on the role of landlord for the thousands of people, they took on the responsibility to provide a safe and healthy living environment for these people.

While no one should have been exposed to a toxin for over two years, I think that the CDC should take advantage of this disaster and learn everything they can about formaldehyde. . . . [T]he fact that no one can tell us how long the effects of formaldehyde will stay with us, is horrifying. This is not a new chemical. There should be more information on it. When the CDC and ATSDR first knew that people were living in these levels and there was even a possibility that they were getting sick, they should have stepped in and found out what was going on. Two years later, after so many people have moved on, some even died in these trailers, it may be too late to know the full extent of what effect formaldehyde has on people. . . . I felt like after it was first known that the formaldehyde was a problem, we were lab rats subjected to the toxin, but no one wanted to record the results.

Editor's note: Lindsay has told me that since living in the FEMA trailer, she has been getting headaches several times a week. She has noticed that exposure to gasoline will trigger a migraine. When her daughter Lelah encounters cigarette smoke, she develops a headache. When Lindsay uses various cleaning products around the house, Lelah says, "That stinks, Mom, I'm going out on the porch." She gets nauseous from these kind of exposures. Exposure to nail polish also makes Lelah feel sick.

H. D.

9/11 Exposure

Looking back, I still find it odd that I never heard the first plane hit. The business I worked in was located on the thirty-third and thirty-fourth floors of a building just across the street from the South Tower of the World Trade Center. We often stopped at the World Trade Center to get coffee in the morning. This particular day most of us had already arrived at the office by 8:45 A.M., but it was only when one of our employees called the office to say a plane had struck the World Trade Center that any of us were aware that anything had happened. We immediately went to the windows to look out at the Twin Towers. As we looked upwards, we could see the gaping hole and the smoke and fire pouring out as we listened to sirens from the police and fire departments. We quickly logged on to the local news channel on our computers to learn more.

While others continued looking at the World Trade Center, I was busy answering the phones that were ringing continuously as people were calling in to see if their husband or wife or friend had made it into the office safely. Suddenly, I heard what sounded like a sonic boom that startled me so much that I jumped and let out a yelp. It was then that the computers and phones went down, followed by the electricity and lights going out. I knew at once that we should vacate the offices. We didn't yet realize that a second plane had hit.

After I assembled everyone who was in the office, we began the descent down the emergency stairs. People were coming into the stairwell from every floor. When we got down to around the eighth floor, we heard a horrible rumbling and thundering echoing in the stairwell, and we could feel the building shaking. People began screaming, but when this happened someone would yell, "Just keep calm and keep going." Everyone continued downward, hastening their pace. When I look back, I believe that the first tower must have collapsed when we heard that awful rumbling as we were making our way down the stairs. When we got to the lobby, everyone there was talking about what they had seen and heard. It was all a buzz. The building manager held a walkie-talkie and told us to exit out the back of the building, proceed south, cut over to the Brooklyn Bridge, and walk over the bridge into Brooklyn.

I took off my jacket before leaving the lobby and put it over my head; I also tied a handkerchief over my nose and mouth. White powder was falling like heavy snow. You couldn't recognize anything, even though you had walked down these same streets a hundred times. Everything was covered ankle deep in the thick white dust. There was pandemonium in the streets. Everyone was running every which way, and you could hear people screaming. Some were just frozen in their tracks, unable to move. It was a horrible scene.

As I was running in a southerly direction as instructed, I heard a terrible rumbling coming from behind me. When I turned around, I saw that the second tower was coming down. People all around me were screaming and scrambling to get away. The cloud of dust that surrounded us began to turn black at this point. I could hardly breathe, and the air burned my mouth. I was unable to see anything, not even a foot in front of myself. All I could think about was getting as far away as I could from the devastation. I saw a woman who was just standing still with a look of horror on her face. I told her to come with me and she did. Later we passed another woman who was obviously in shock. She was sobbing and kept repeating that she knew people who worked in the World Trade Center Towers. I told her to come with us and she did. The three of us continued running to the southern tip of Manhattan, where the dust clouds weren't so black. We stopped to regain our composure amid the blaring sirens. Just about everyone around us was talking on their cell phones. One guy reported that the Pentagon had been hit and also the Sears Tower in Chicago. The latter was of course just a false rumor.

Hours later I finally made it home to Staten Island. When I turned on my television, I could not believe my eyes. To think that I was in the middle of that! While listening to the broadcast in a state of stunned disbelief, I took off my dust-coated clothes and put them in a bag along with my fabric purse and its contents. I double bagged my clothes and put them in the garbage. When I took a shower, I scrubbed myself thoroughly, but when I dried off, I still felt slimy. I had to take three showers before my skin felt normal again.

About three or four days later, I began coughing. Once I would start I didn't seem to be able to stop. My whole chest was aching as a result.

My hands and feet were swollen considerably, and the swelling got worse and worse as the days passed. I couldn't touch the skin on my hands or feet without feeling extreme pain. The sensitivity to touch became so acute that I couldn't bear it any longer and went to get medical attention. I could barely stand up and walk. Just getting out of the house was a real challenge. I couldn't stand to let anything touch my skin; even a puff of wind across my skin was too much to bear. My coughing and difficulty in breathing continued to be an issue as well. Tests showed that I had developed severe asthma, which I had never had in the past. At first, the doctors were unable to determine what was causing the swelling and sensitivity of my hands and feet. Then weeks of extensive testing indicated that I had suffered arsenic poisoning. This arsenic exposure had produced nerve damage to my hands and feet that resulted in a very painful sensitivity to touch. Even with the ever-increasing doses of painkillers that I was given, I could barely walk or dress myself. I remained inactive during this period because I couldn't use my hands and feet. I was unable to continue working and had to go on welfare after I had exhausted my personal savings.

Doctors told me that over time the arsenic would leave my system. Although the levels have diminished, it has taken almost five years, and residual effects still linger. I did begin to slowly regain the use of my hands and could once again walk, albeit short distances for brief periods of time. To this day, the use of my hands has been dramatically affected. As a result of my reduced capacities, it has been extremely difficult for me to continue in the same type of work I had been doing for the past fifteen years. The loss of income has been particularly difficult, especially with all the medical bills to cover. Since the damage to my nerves cannot be reversed, I will remain very limited in my ability to walk any distance and to use my hands at work. Additionally, my asthma continues to be a problem, and I now experience asthma attacks when I encounter various chemical odors. But how can one avoid chemicals and still lead a normal life? I still cannot believe that I have been so disabled because of the 9/11 attack and am in such poor health now, when I was never sick before, not even with a cold.

Capt. Richard Caron

Gulf War Veteran

Before I went to the Gulf War, I had a full-time job as a carpenter. I was also the pastor of a Baptist church and the chaplain of my Army National Guard unit. My health was good before I went to the Persian Gulf.

My unit arrived in Saudi Arabia in early December and soon moved northwest to our desert camp about fifteen miles from the border of Iraq. When the air war started, chemical alarms went off many times. This was the point at which we were given the pyridostigmine bromide pills because they were supposed to be an anti-nerve gas medication. Within a few days, I wasn't feeling well; I was fatigued, had headaches, and muscle and joint aches. At this time, I was so busy doing lots of different things that I thought I was having health problems because I was on the go for what seemed like twenty-four hours a day. Within a few weeks, however, I started noticing that diesel exhaust and the fumes from diesel fuel were making me slightly nauseated, even though I had been around diesel before the war without any problem.

When the ground war started, I went forward with my company to a position only five miles from the Iraqi border. We had one SCUD missile explode about seven or eight miles from us. When Saddam Hussein gave orders to set all the oil wells on fire, the air was so full of smoke that daytime was like nighttime. We were close enough to the fires that we could see the flames and hear the roar of the fires. The smoke started bothering me a lot.

The insect spray we were using was also bothering me. My skin would get red when I used it. By this point, I was often getting short of breath—I didn't know whether that was from the fires or the insect repellant. I had bronchitis several times while I was in the Persian Gulf. Before we left Saudi Arabia, we were given a physical. My blood pressure was really high, 180/104. Before I went to the Gulf War, it had been 120/70.

In June 1991, I was released from active duty. A week later I ended up going to the Veterans' Administration hospital in my state. I was having a hard time breathing, and I had bronchitis again. I told the doctors there about the various other symptoms I was also having. By this point I was getting sick from household cleaning products, and going into a store would make me sick. Before the Gulf War, I had only had a couple of migraines, but I started having them all the time during the war, and they continued when I returned to the States.

Since my health problems continued for a year or two, the local VA hospital finally sent me to the VA hospital in Washington, D.C. There they diagnosed me with chronic fatigue syndrome, asthma, sleep apnea, and brain damage (the brain damage was shown on an MRI). My hands and arms would also sometimes go numb, and they told me I had carpal tunnel syndrome. I'd never had that before the war, however. While I was at the VA hospital in Washington, I met other Gulf War vets who had symptoms similar to mine and were also sensitive to chemicals at this point. Through them I learned about a doctor at a VA hospital in Northhampton, Massachusetts, who was very interested in multiple chemical sensitivity. About six months after I left Washington, I entered the Northhampton hospital, where they kept me for three months and I was diagnosed with MCS. They sent me to a VA hospital in Connecticut to have a SPECT scan. It showed damage to my right frontal lobe and right temple, as well as damage to the right side of my thalamus.

I have had to make many adjustments in my life because of the chemical sensitivity I had brought back from the Gulf War. I had to give up my job as pastor at my church because I was having a hard time remembering scripture passages that I used to know by heart.

Because the construction trade was slow at the time I returned from the war, I got a job in law enforcement because I had previous experience in the field. I worked for the sheriff's department for a while and also for a city police department. I wasn't able to continue that line of work, however, because I had become very forgetful since my return from the war and would get confused about where I was. There would be times when I'd be out driving on roads that I'd traveled many times before, and sometimes I couldn't remember where I was. I would just have to keep going, and finally I would realize where I was. When I was trying to work in law enforcement, I would get a call to go to a certain location where something was happening, and I couldn't remember where that street was located. So I just had to give up that work.

Before I went to the Gulf War, I used to love to go snowmobiling, but I can't go anymore because the diesel exhaust fumes give me a headache and make me feel nauseated. My sensitivity to chemicals makes life pretty difficult. Perfume bothers me, and so do newspapers and magazines. I get nausea and headaches from the ink, and my nose gets stuffed up. I broke out in rashes while I was in Desert Storm, and I still get rashes today. I have a lot of problem with asthma now, and I didn't have asthma before the war.

MCS also affects your home life a lot. It's hard on my wife to have me be so sensitive to chemicals now. When I left for the war, I was in good health. Now my health is bad, and I never feel like myself, I never feel good. I don't feel like going places my wife wants to go, and many places I can't go because people are wearing perfume. Sometimes I have to wear a mask to go in a store, and I feel like people are staring at me when I wear it.

At first I was having a hard time getting compensation from the government when I filed claims on different things I had been diagnosed with. They kept turning me down. Then finally they used some other diagnoses so I could get some disability payments. I'm now getting 100% compensation because I can't work. I had to keep pushing and pushing to get that money. I just wouldn't give up, and the Disabled American Veterans Association helped me out a lot. It took me seven years to get that full disability status from the Veterans' Administration. In the meantime I had applied for Social Security disability in 1996, and I got that in seven months.

I've noticed that the younger servicemen who are Gulf War vets are reluctant to let people know that they're not feeling well. Many of them are still on active duty, and they're afraid that if they let anyone know that they're sick, they will be discharged.

The VA hospitals are still just treating symptoms, but they haven't come up with any cure. I think it's a terrible shame the way they are treating the Gulf War vets, but it's no surprise to me because they treated the Vietnam vets who were exposed to Agent Orange the same way.

Phyllis "Dolly" La Joie

Exxon Valdez Cleanup Worker

When I heard that the *Exxon Valdez* had run aground on a reef in Prince William Sound and that thousands of workers would be needed to help clean up the beaches, I decided to go help. I had spent years in Prince William Sound seal hunting in the commercial fishing industry, and I loved the area. I had also worked in Valdez during the construction of the oil pipeline that carried oil down to the terminal camp, where it was loaded onto tankers for shipment. The building I worked in contained blueprints and documents for the maintenance of the pipeline and pumping stations. I was sort of like a librarian and would help engineers find the blueprints they needed. Once in a while we went out with the engineers to be sure they were building things according to specifications, but it was very cold, so we didn't go with them very often. After the construction of the line, I worked for a while at Prudhoe Bay as an engineering aid. Anyway, I felt guilty that I had helped get the oil from Prudhoe Bay to Valdez, so I thought I should go help clean it up.

About Memorial Day weekend, I signed up in Anchorage with VECO, the company Exxon hired to handle the cleanup. I was told to report around 11 P.M., and we all got on buses for the trip to Valdez, which took all night. It was very hard to sleep sitting up, and the drivers played loud music all night. By the time we arrived in Valdez, we were just exhausted.

When we finally got on the ship to go out to the spill site, it took us over eight hours to get out there because of the rough weather and icebergs. All our living quarters were on barges on the water because there were no clearings on the shores, which were just wild, rocky forested shores. On the long trip out to the *Greens Creek* barge, the barge where I stayed, we bounced, bounced, bounced on these hard benches, so we couldn't sleep.

By the time we arrived, I was absolutely exhausted because I had not had any sleep for two days and a night. But as soon as I got off the boat, they put me to work that night in decontamination. Starting then, I worked a twelve-hour shift every night, seven days a week. We were supposed to occasionally go home for R&R, but we all resisted doing that because the trip back and forth was so long and grueling that it was hardly worth it. To make matters worse, since I worked all night every night, I had to sleep during the day. It wasn't easy to sleep during the day, however, because there were helicopters landing very frequently right on the roof of our living quarters. Everyone in the government from the EPA to Coast Guard officials to Alaskan officials came out to see the spill. They all came to our barge because we had the only helicopter landing pad on Prince William Sound. Our barge also had a medical facility where the injured were brought. So if you worked the night shift and had to sleep during the day, like I did, it was really hard to sleep with all those helicopters coming and going.

Anyway, decontamination (decon) was a crucial part of the whole operation because the workers would return from the beaches covered in oil. When they got off the boat that brought them back to the *Greens Creek* barge, they first stepped onto a big floating platform that was attached to the decon barge, which was in turn attached to the *Greens Creek*. All the workers who got off the boat that brought them back from working all day on the beaches had to drop everything that was covered with oil onto the decon barge. Even though they had been hosed off a certain amount before they left the beaches, they still had lots of oil left on them. So they dropped their life jackets and rain outfits and gloves and boots on the decon barge, everything except their insulated underwear and their coveralls. Their coveralls were supposed to have stayed clean under their outer rain jackets and pants, but they didn't. Even though it was usually cold when the cleanup workers left the *Greens Creek* barge early in the morning to head for the beach, once they started doing heavy work in the hot sun, they would take off their rain gear, so some of them ended up with oil on their coveralls. Those were washed in a laundromat on the barge. At any rate, we decon workers had the job of cleaning during the night all the oily rain jackets and pants and stuff the workers had removed when they returned from work that day.

One job in decon was to use steam guns to steam the oil off the rubber things like the boots and the hard hats, rain pants, rain jackets, and life jackets—anything that you couldn't put in the washing machines. We would lay all these things out on this big flat deck and spray the oil off. Sometimes you would get really tired standing and spraying, and sometimes you would get tired bending down to turn over the rain jackets and other things so you could spray the other side. Sometimes you would get tired of the job of hanging these things up so they would be dry by morning. Because it was so cold and wet at night, the rain gear and boots had to be dried in these things that were like boxcars that contained blowers and heaters. We took turns doing most of the jobs, and everybody worked together really well.

We were supposed to use goggles because of the oily water that was splashing all around us and the oily steam that filled the air when we were steaming the oil off the rain gear and boots. But the goggles would get steamed up really fast, especially if you were down on the deck turning the rain gear to the other side. After a while, we started realizing that we were getting chemicals steamed into our lungs, and we thought, boy, this isn't good. In orientation, they had told us about all the chemicals that are found in crude oil. Here we were steaming it and breathing in the oily mist, so we thought we had better take some precautions. We tried respirators for a while, but we couldn't get enough and ran out in a couple of weeks or so. The suppliers couldn't keep up with the demand for gloves or respirators.

We washed the oily coveralls and underwear in a washing machine. We used Tide at first, but then they started sending us some strong solvents to add because it was really hard to get the oil out of everything. They wanted to make sure that not one drop of oil got onto the berthing vessel where we slept, so we used some pretty strong stuff that worked better. It was industrial-strength stuff. I don't remember all the names, but one product we used was Simple Green. The laundry room, which held just one washer and dryer, was small, and the vapor made me sick a lot of the time. When you washed the oily clothes and dried them in the dryer, you had oil vapor everywhere, and it was a strong smell. Sometimes I felt like I was drunk and was going to pass out. Then I would have to go outside to get away from the fumes and get some fresh air. Whenever it was really cold, as it often was at night, we would have to keep the laundry room door shut to keep from freezing. Then the fumes were really thick.

We had to wash a lot of loads every night, so we kept the machines going all the time. The beach workers ran out of gloves fast, like right away, because they had each been issued just five pairs. That's why we started washing the gloves instead of throwing them away, which we had been told to do in orientation. We didn't have much of a choice because the suppliers couldn't keep up with our needs. The workers had to have gloves, and we didn't have any new gloves to give them. A few gloves had separate liners, but most were stiff, heavy, thick, lined gloves, men's work gloves made out of rubber or plastic. After we put the gloves through the washer, we had to turn them inside out before we put them in the dryer so that the cloth lining would dry. You had to put them on your hand so you could turn them inside out and pull the lining out to dry them. Then after they were dry, they had to be turned right-side-out again.

Turning the gloves ended up being my job because no one else would do it. The young girls wouldn't do it because they were afraid it would break their fingernails and ruin them like mine were from all the solvents and the oil. When you tried to pull out the lining, you could feel it in every tendon of your arm and across your shoulders. It was an excruciating job, but it had to be done because the workers had to have gloves. Anyway, whenever there were gloves to be turned, everyone else disappeared. Sometimes I turned gloves practically the whole night. I have tendonitis now in my hands, wrists, shoulders, in my back. Oh, man, I cried some nights because my hands hurt so bad. One day my hands were so swollen I couldn't even get dressed or open the door of my unit. The doctor bound my hands to reduce the swelling. I have pictures of that. Fortunately, I was able to go on R&R for a week right after that, which helped my hands.

About this time, I think it was in July, they needed more people for the beach cleanup, so I started working on the beaches. I was eager to get out on the beaches because I thought I would get some fresh air that way by getting away from those fumes in that little laundry room. Besides, my hands couldn't take the glove turning any longer. I also liked the idea of working during the day so I could sleep at night when the helicopters weren't landing.

Well, I didn't get much fresh air on the beaches after all. The smell on the beaches was awful, like something dead. Crude oil has a sickening odor all its own. It's horrible. Of course, we found dead things, too, like seals and birds. If we found something dead, we had to call up the Coast Guard and tell them we had found an animal so they could send somebody over to pick it up. We would put the dead seals or birds in plastic bags. It was pretty sickening to have to pick up these animals and birds that had been decomposing for several months.

The whole beach scene was wild, with people jumping from boat to boat and from rocks to the shore, with slippery oil covering everything. It was just a world of constant falls and slips. It was really hard on our knees and feet. We were given thin rubber deck boots that protected us from the oil but not from injury. This stuff was unbelievable. It was really dangerous and dirty work. They didn't think a woman should be doing it, especially a small one like me, but I showed them I could do it.

My first day on the beaches the crew initiated me by turning on full blast this high-pressure steam gun that I was holding, and it flipped me over. We sprayed the oil-covered rocks with these steam guns and also with cold water from high-pressure hoses. Using these big pressure hoses was hard, hard work because that high pressure is hard to hold down. You couldn't let go because you could almost kill someone if you did. So you put the hose over your shoulder and put it under your arm to move it because the high pressure made it so hard to control.

We had been told in orientation that whenever we were using the steam guns on oil-covered rocks or were around the oil fumes we should wear a respirator because of the fumes. But when we asked our foreman why we couldn't get respirators, he said, "Well, you can go home if you don't want to do it." He couldn't get respirators for us, so I usually just wore one of those little paper masks. But of course that paper mask didn't do much to keep me from breathing in a lot of that oily mist that surrounded us as we sprayed steam on the oily rocks.

The oil was everywhere—it was three feet deep in some places—and it was slippery. You had to crawl in it every time you fell, so you ended up with it all over you. Even though we tried to tape up the gaps between our gloves and our boots and our rain gear, the oil just ate away at the tape and the edges opened up between your gloves and your boots and your rain gear. No matter how tight you sealed yourself up, the oil would still seep in. In the mornings it was freezing cold, so you'd wear all these clothes, but by noon, it was like being in a sauna. You would start stripping off layers, and sometimes you would end up working in just your life jacket and coveralls and underwear, so all those things would get sprayed with the oily mist that was coming off the rocks as you sprayed them. I got a lot of oil on my skin and on my face. A couple of times I even got oil in my eyes. In orientation they told us we should wear special full-body protective suits while we were working around the oil. We were supposed to wear these suits every day, but I never saw them on the beaches.

After I finished working on the oil spill in September of 1989, I spent a little time in Anchorage and then returned to my sister's home in Hawaii to help her for the winter. I ended up living there for a number of years until I moved to Wisconsin to be closer to my daughter. I didn't even start looking for a job until January of 1990 because I was so exhausted from all those long hours of work on the oil spill, twelve hours a day, seven days a week for over three months, with only one or two weeks off for R&R. When I did try to work, I would get really tired before the end of a shift, so I tried doing part-time work. At first I tried to work nights at a duty-free shop. Then that summer I worked as a census taker so I could be outside. I kept having colds all the time, just like when I was working on the spill. (It was called the Valdez Crud.) I also started having sinus problems in Hawaii, and that had never happened to me before in that warm, humid climate.

I continued feeling really tired if I worked too long or too hard, but I could handle a job as long as I didn't have to use my brain. For some reason, I just couldn't get my brain functioning in the morning. Then in December of 1991, I got very sick with some kind of a sinus infection or something and started running a temperature. I couldn't get my temperature down. I would stay home and rest and start to feel better so I could go back to work for a day. Then, whammo, I would end up in bed again. I thought I had some kind of horrible flu. Antibiotics were no help, and this went on for months. Finally, I took some time off under temporary disability insurance and discovered I felt better if I didn't exert myself too often.

During this period, I felt like my head was going to explode. It's hard to explain, and it didn't feel quite like a sinus headache. The pressure would just be so bad that I had to crawl to the bathroom. It was excruciating, and this went on for months. My Kaiser doctor said he couldn't figure out what was wrong. I also started having bad stomach problems in December of 1991—severe nausea in the morning and terrible bloating.

I tried desperately to find some kind of work that I could handle even though I was feeling so awful. For a while, I worked three hours a day as a companion to an elderly doctor with Alzheimer's. But just getting ready and driving over there and sitting with him, fixing him a sandwich, and going home would wipe me out for the rest of the day. Then as his Alzheimer's progressed, I had to give up that job because I couldn't work full time like they wanted. I also worked for some other patients, but eventually I became too ill to even do that, so I went on welfare. I just couldn't do anything else.

Eventually, my doctor diagnosed me with diabetes and found that my liver was enlarged. The medication he gave me for the diabetes did help a lot, but I still wasn't able to function in the morning. To make matters worse, my doctor suggested that I could work full time if I wanted to. When I applied for Social Security disability payments, I was even sent to a psychiatrist, who told me he thought I was delusional about some of my health problems.

A friend who had worked with me on the oil spill had sent me a newspaper article some time back about cleanup workers getting sick. I didn't pay any attention to it, however, because we hadn't been told what symptoms to watch for or anything like that. I had no idea that the health problems I had developed since working on the cleanup could be from the oil exposures. Then one day one of my former co-workers in the oil spill cleanup that I hadn't talked to in a long time called me to see how I was doing. I told her that I had been in bed sick for quite a while. She said that they were all getting sick and said I should get tested for the chemicals we had been exposed to during the cleanup. So I had my blood tested, and the results showed elevated levels of several of those chemicals. My doctor didn't know anything about chemical poisoning, however. He referred me to an industrial doctor, who also didn't know much about chemical poisoning. Fortunately, I at last found a physician who was familiar with cases in which people had developed chemical sensitivity.

When my health started really going downhill in December of 1991, I developed a lot of other problems. I have hardly any hair left. On my back I've got these odd things that are like big brown moles. Some are constant, and some come and go. My doctor doesn't know what they are. My fingernails are rotting off. I used to have an excellent memory, but that's no longer true. I can't remember the names of a lot of the people that I worked with cleaning up the spill, and I thought I would never forget them. I can't do math anymore, and I used to be a math whiz.

Sometimes I just completely lose feeling and drop things. Not too long ago I tried to lift a black iron skillet. Nothing happened. If I write too much or if I lift heavy things, I get stiffness and tingling in my hands. If I get overtired, I ache all over, and sometimes I have trouble getting up out of a chair. I should never have held those high-pressure hoses all day long during the cleanup.

Various chemical exposures bother me since I got sick after working on the oil spill. Traffic exhaust gives me a headache and makes me nauseated. Cigarette smoke and certain cleaning products and perfumes make me choke and cough, give me a headache, and make me sick to my stomach. One day when I walked by a shop that sells thongs and rubber slippers, like everyone wears in Hawaii, the rubber smell made me throw up.

I've been diagnosed with COPD (chronic obstructive pulmonary disease), gallstones, and severe anemia. Now I also have asthma, and sometimes I cough so much that I can hardly talk. Recently I've been bothered a lot by vertigo, so I had an MRI. It didn't explain the vertigo, but it did show that I have an aneurism in my brain.

Helping to clean up the oil spill seemed like the right thing to do in 1989, but now that my cleanup work has ruined my health, I wish I had stayed in Hawaii instead of returning to Alaska to help clean the beaches.

Jenn Duncan

9/11 Brooklyn Resident

Things were going well in my life until the fall of 2000. In 1992, I had graduated from MIT, where I got a degree in a joint venture between humanities and science. I studied some biochemistry and electrical engineering, and I also studied media arts. Then I went on to get a master's from NYU in interactive telecommunications. At the time, the web was developing, so for me it was the perfect mix of technology and creativity, the perfect blend at the perfect time at the perfect place. I worked for many years in New York City in the multimedia field. One of my favorite projects was a website for Children's Television Workshop, which produces "Sesame Street." I also worked for Viacom and a number of other companies. My plan was to pay off my loans and then go back to school for a doctorate in the biomedical field, so I studied medical and neurology material in preparation for that goal.

Life was also good outside of my work. My activities included dance and a movement technique called Continuum that's like yoga combined with other things, and I was qualifying to be a teacher of Continuum. I was in great shape physically and kept a healthy balance in my life. I liked to travel and had taken advanced scuba diving. Outings in the city with friends for dinner, theater, museums, concerts, and movies were an important part of my life. Drumming was one of the activities that I loved. African drumming was a special interest because I grew up in Africa as the daughter of teachers working there with humanitarian services.

Then all that changed when I was thirty-two after my office building installed a new carpet in a poorly ventilated area adjacent to one of my primary working areas. Painting and other renovations made the situation worse. It wasn't long before I got very ill and found it difficult to sleep. I suffered from headaches and had unusual pain in the back of my head. Nausea was a problem and made it difficult for me to eat; I felt like I had a bad case of the flu all of the time and had difficulty breathing. Within several weeks, everything just started disintegrating. I was walking into walls, falling a lot, and dropping things. In the middle of conversations, I would blank out and not realize what was happening for several minutes. My sense of space was so impaired that even now I get disoriented in new buildings. It takes several repeat visits until I can grasp a basic sense of rooms and halls and doorways.

I was getting lost on my way to work where I had traveled every weekday for over a year. I would get lost in my own neighborhood just trying to go to the bank that was only two blocks away. Sometimes I couldn't find my way home for a few hours. When that happened, I would sit and rest and move a few more feet and sit and rest and try to figure out which way I needed to go.[1]

With the mounting evidence, my doctors realized these problems were most likely the result of chemical injury. Later on I was diagnosed with CBI (chemical brain injury), a type of TBI (traumatic brain injury) that produces effects like those of strokes. I had damage to my pre-frontal lobe, slowed thinking, memory problems, and a significant IQ drop. My speech became slurred, and I stuttered and had trouble finding words.

Exposure to cologne or traffic exhaust or somebody smoking a cigarette would produce extreme disorientation, trouble breathing, and excruciating joint pain, all of which made it very difficult for me to move or think. It was less than a year after I developed this chemical sensitivity that the 9/11 attacks occurred. With all that toxic smoke drifting across the river into Brooklyn during the months that the pile burned, my symptoms got worse. My absent-mindedness and physical limitations

---

[1] Editor's note: Staff Sergeant Pat Browning, who drove a tractor-trailer truck during the 1991 Gulf War, came home with Gulf War syndrome. Like so many other sick Gulf War veterans, she too experienced severe memory loss. Her story in my book *Gulf War Syndrome: Legacy of a Perfect War* contains this passage:

> When I first came back from the war, I had a lot of problems remembering things. One day I drove my kids to school and dropped them off, but then instead of driving home I just wandered around for a couple of hours because I couldn't remember where I was going.

made it very difficult and dangerous for me to leave my apartment, and I became homebound.

On one occasion, a month or two after 9/11, when the fires were still burning and the smoke was sometimes drifting our direction, I was in downtown Brooklyn trying to go shopping for some food when I started to collapse and had to sit down on the curb doubled over. I had no choice but to give up on my shopping trip and try and get home before I completely lost my ability to function and know where I was. With great difficulty, I succeeded in hailing a car service (Brooklyn's version of a taxi), but I had a lot of trouble explaining to the driver where I needed to go. I couldn't speak and couldn't figure out how to use money or make change or pay him. I don't remember how I made it back.

As my condition kept deteriorating, life became hellish. I would sleep a few hours, wake up in pain, force myself to get a drink of water or go to the bathroom or perform some task necessary for survival, and then collapse in exhaustion. Even though I was deeply exhausted, I could not fall asleep for hours because of the pain and my hyperactive mind. Finally, I might get a few hours of sleep, but I never felt rested. Waking meant more pain, and it took hours before I could get my body to respond enough for me to move. There was no sense of day or night, no regularity for sleep or eating at all. Along with all my physical problems, my extreme short-term memory loss made ordinary activities almost impossible. I could not retain things in my mind for more than a few seconds.[2]

I would get up and think OK, today I have to take a shower. It would then take me a couple of hours to get my body moving. By that time, I would have forgotten what I was going to do. Maybe a few days later I would get it together enough to actually take a shower. Because taking a shower in my condition was dangerous, I had to muster as much strength as I could. It was such a slow process to organize everything. One day maybe I would remember to get my clothes out, but even that

---

[2] Dr. Jill Bolte Taylor, a neuroanatomist who suffered a massive stroke, describes her experience in a talk titled "My Stroke of Insight" she gave at the annual Technology, Entertainment, Design (TED) conference in 2006. A video of her speech may be seen at www.ted.com/index.php/speakers/view/id/203.

was difficult because of my joint pain and because I had trouble remembering what I was doing. A couple of days later I might manage to get out some towels. Then I made sure I rested really well the day or two before my actual shower. I could only do this about once a month because it was so hard.

When I would finally take my shower, I had to really pay attention to what I was doing. I had to sit down on the floor of the tub under the shower because I was too weak and shaky to try to stand up. It would take a long time to wash myself because I could not lift my arms very far; raising them all the way up to wash my hair was almost impossible. I had to rest and coax myself along, rest and coax. My lungs would hurt worse and worse because the hot moist air was hard on them. It felt like I could not get enough air.

After I was done with my shower, I would be in a lot more pain and could hardly sit up. The exertion wiped me out so much that I could not get myself out of the tub and had to lie there for maybe an hour. Once I passed out in the water and came to choking and gasping for air. After that experience, I started hooking my arm over the side of the tub so that I wouldn't slip down into the water and drown. (Poor drainage meant there were several inches of standing water in the tub.) It made my arm hurt, but it kept me from drowning. When I would finally get enough strength together to get out of the tub, I could only lie on the bathroom floor for a while. It took a huge effort to grab a towel to cover myself so I wouldn't freeze. I would have to lie there for another hour or two before I could manage to get back to my bedroom. Sometimes I would stay on the bathroom floor all night because I didn't have the strength to drag myself out of the bathroom.

Getting enough to eat was also very hard. I was having trouble figuring out how to do things in the kitchen. If a pot was dirty, I couldn't figure out what to do about it. I couldn't figure out what I was supposed to do, how to clean it or to just use something else. I would have to sit there and chant in my head, "scrub the pot with the yellow sponge, scrub the pot with the yellow sponge, and then get the beans." I would have to make these chants and just repeat them, drill them into my head over and over and over before finally the plan would stick at least a little and I could try to carry it out. Because of the muscle and joint pain, every motion would burn and hurt and make my body sore for hours with no relief. From the time I started feeling hungry, it would often take me six hours or more to get some kind of food into my body. Even then, it was often old, burned, and not well varied. Some days I could not manage to eat at all.

Having a cat helped motivate me sometimes because he would be hungry and noisy, so I would finally drag myself to the kitchen to find him some food. Then I would just sit on the floor with the fridge door open, trying to make sense of the shapes and things. If something was behind something else, forget it. There was no way I could grasp in my mind that there were things in the back of the fridge out of sight.

Everything was becoming rather hopeless, and that was the kind of struggle that I was enduring at home every day. I was walking into walls and falling, but I wasn't able to communicate and tell anybody that I was having such problems. If somebody called and left a message, I couldn't figure out how to return a call, how to write down the phone number or get it from the machine. It seemed very strange that I had gone from building electronics and programming software to not understanding how to use a phone or e-mail.

It was like that for long blocks of time and would get worse after they sprayed for the West Nile virus. At first I didn't know that's what was happening; I would just suddenly notice that my condition had deteriorated. Finally, I figured out that my symptoms would get worse when they sprayed, so whenever that happened, I would try to close all the windows if I had the strength and would turn my air filters up.

Sometimes when I was in a really bad state, I felt like I was in a bubble, a blue heavy bubble so dense that I couldn't get through. And I kept thinking, I've been used to communicating well in my past. I kept trying to puzzle out how to communicate and to figure out how to say things, but I couldn't capture the sense of what I meant into words. If I did remember a key word or phrase, I couldn't retain it in my neurocircuits for even a few seconds, especially in the middle of a conversation. The demands of listening, interpreting, remembering points, choosing answers, finding words, working the mechanisms of one's voice, and finally speaking in the proper rhythm and accepted social context are more highly demanding than any of us consciously realize. I just had to keep waiting for my body to catch up with what my mind wanted to express. It's taken years for me to regain some oral facility, and my speech abilities still have not fully returned. I have to prepare for common ordinary events well in advance, and rehearse over and over what is to be expected and what I am supposed to do or say. Sometimes with preparation I can fake it for a short time, but often simple exchanges and conversations fall apart in disaster.

During the time when I was in the worst condition, I lost the ability to read and write, but over a long time I was able to retrain myself to do that to some extent. I could sound out an individual word, but I could not remember it long enough for a phrase or sentence to have any meaning. I would "read" an article about chemical injury and know it was relevant, but I could not make any use of the information because I could retain it for only a few seconds. By contrast, before I developed multiple chemical sensitivity, I would memorize Shakespeare speeches for fun.

I had started turning the TV on at night when I was in pain and alone just to have the company of a human voice and to distract myself from the agony. Eventually, I used television to help regain my ability to listen and hear and pay attention to others' speech. I spent months, almost a year, just listening to television so that I could eventually comprehend people again. When real people would talk, I would hear only pieces of what they said. By the time they finished a sentence, I could no longer remember what they had said at the beginning and I could not figure out how to reply, especially in time.

I could not tolerate television at first, it was too complicated with too much overwhelming visual sensations and loud sounds. To retrain my mind, I spent months and months just listening to Sesame Street and other children's programs. Later on I would sometimes watch a few minutes of high school education courses about subjects like math and biology and history. Although I could not understand them or solve the problems, I knew the diagrams looked familiar. I had some inner sense that if I just let these things exist in my environment, eventually I might reconnect to some of them.

Much later on I tried watching the news, and I was only able to do this in an unusual way. First, I had to relearn how to work the remote. I spent a month or two hitting play and rewind and record, learning how to work the VCR. This was a sharp contrast to the days when I was building devices and writing manuals for that kind of thing. After I figured out how to work the remote again, I would record the news and then play one sentence at a time and then rewind and play it again. I would repeat in my head what I had just heard. If I could not repeat it,

I would rewind again and listen to the same little clip. I would listen to the same sentence over and over again until I could say what it was I had heard. I would often fall asleep for a while because the effort was so exhausting. It would take me hours or days to watch the half-hour evening news in this way.

Years later I still cannot comprehend radio because people speak faster on radio than on TV, and the captioning on the TV helps me follow along.

It took a few years before I got to the point where I could write a letter to someone or fill out some forms so that people would start to understand what was happening to me. I still have a lot of trouble expressing things in writing and need a lot of assistance. Finally, I was able to get some social services and a health aide for several hours a day. It was such a relief when the health aide came. It meant that instead of just eating one meal every day or two, I was able to eat a couple of times a day. The weight of all that wasn't on me. The first time that I took a bath, the health aide sat right outside. She said, "I'm gong to sit here. It's my job to sit here and make sure you're safe in the water." I broke down in tears because it was such a relief to finally not have to put so much effort into keeping super-alert right when I was most exhausted and weak and not being so afraid that I might fall or slip under the water. I'll never forget that feeling of relief; it was a little piece of heaven. My health aides are my guardian angels. Literally, they helped save my life, and I am deeply grateful to them.

I depend on my health aides for shopping, for taking something to the mail, for little errands, for just about everything because I'm pretty much homebound now. I use a wheelchair or walker. When I do have to go out to see a doctor, I wear a mask because of the auto exhaust I encounter on the way and all the disinfectants, ammonia, chlorine, fragrances, and petroleum-based products I run into at the clinic. Those kinds of exposures give me breathing difficulties and neurological reactions. I get headaches, get confused and disoriented, and have great difficulty paying attention and understanding things. My muscle coordination and strength deteriorates, my spasms and twitching get stronger, and I develop very bad joint and muscle pain. Eventually, I lose the ability to move, and my body gets totally paralyzed for several hours. In these situations, I attempt to use a respirator mask, but I can only breathe through it for an hour or two before it gets difficult to inhale because my lungs aren't as strong as they used to be. Sometimes I have started to black out and have had to call an emergency crew to get oxygen, so now I take along my own tank whenever I'm out.

On one occasion, I arranged to go to a doctor's appointment in an ambulette, which is a wheelchair-accessible van. I wore my mask, but the ambulette contained several air fresheners. When I asked the driver to remove them, he did, but the scent had soaked into the upholstery and the seats. It got on my coat and all my things. I started having a headache and getting disoriented, and by the time I got to the doctor's I was having heavy spasms and twitches. As a result, I was really struggling to talk and explain the things that I needed to discuss with the doctor.

To make matters worse, on the way back home, the ambulette took a detour to pick up somebody else. When he made this stop, the driver left the back door open and diesel fumes poured in. At that point, I went limp and keeled over with a major headache and had to vomit. Luckily, my aide managed to grab a bag in time, but it was just horrendous. I could no longer speak or move my limbs. On the way back home, I was experiencing spasms that caused me to jerk all around. When we finally arrived, I was unable to move. My aide had to get me inside on her own, get the contaminated clothes off me, get me into bed, and leave some finger food and water nearby before she left. I lay there unable to speak, move, eat or do anything for hours.

Of course, I had known that after a trip like this I would often feel really sick for two or three days afterwards and have spasms and jerk a lot, and not really recover for two to three weeks at least. Usually after any trip out, I get complete muscular paralysis by the next day and can't move a single muscle for hours. My health aide has gotten very good at watching for me to twitch a finger or eyelid so that she knows I'm conscious. I cough and cough, usually producing lots of fluid, but I can't even roll myself onto my side so I won't choke. When I begin to emerge from that state, if I need water I might go "Wahhh, wahhh, wahhh," and my aide knows what I mean. There's a whole sign language we've worked out.

Sometimes it's hard to think that I used to be capable of doing things like calculus and differential equations. Now if somebody asks me numbers or to spell something, it's really hard. I have dyslexia sometimes. I always check and double-check when I write something because letters would be returned because I had mixed up my numbers. All this is frustrating because I have a degree from MIT and from NYU. A lot of the multimedia projects I used to work on were somehow connected to education. That was something that meant a lot to me. I also wanted to obtain a Ph.D. in the biomedical field. And now instead of being a contributor to society, I have to depend on help from Social Security and health aides. I can't build and do things and create and give back the way that I could before I became chemically sensitive, and that's hard for me to take. Most of my limited energy goes to survival and very simple, basic needs.

In 2006, my landlord attempted to evict me, and despite my doctor's strong objections, an advocacy agency tried to force me to move into an extremely toxic apartment that would have endangered my health and life. Although I tried very hard, I could not arrange things, write, communicate, or advocate for myself properly because of my injuries.

At last, a kind person who also was chemically sensitive and had seen me on the documentary *The Toxic Clouds of 9/11* came to my rescue and helped me locate a suitable small house a couple of hours north of New York. A compassionate couple who had also seen me on the documentary helped with various legal matters and packed up my things and drove me to my new place. My health improved somewhat in this cleaner atmosphere, but relocating has disrupted the regular patterns I had reestablished. My functionality was reduced again, and I had to slowly relearn and reconnect to many simple processes such as finding stores that carry the special foods I need, changing my address, and getting my house organized. Although I have been able to find health aides here, who are again my guardian angels, I have been unable to access other critically needed services and agencies despite a year of trying and applying. I still need extensive help with writing and communicating, which keeps me from handling crucial legal or social-service matters in a timely fashion.

Even more alarming, it seems that the general lack of awareness of chemical brain injury and chemical injury and my considerable medical needs will soon force me to move once again. This is a terrifying prospect because my chemical sensitivity makes it extremely difficult to find a place to live that my body can tolerate, and my physical weakness makes it impossible to do the labor of moving. It would take another huge effort to search for a medically acceptable location and organize a move. The timing and strain also jeopardizes all that I have rebuilt this year and all the other urgent needs I must deal with immediately or risk losing critical medical, social service, and legal resources. Although I will try the best I can, without some kind of assistance I am afraid I won't have the strength to handle this again.

Thank you to my mother for helping keep me alive until my aides came. I am also especially thankful for the support from some understanding and compassionate people. Even an act that seems small to a healthy person can make a huge difference to someone with impairments. I remain always grateful for the progress I have made and for the chance to be alive.

Editor's note: Jenn wishes to thank AJ, TJ, JM, and SB for assistance in writing this story. Most of it is a transcription from the footage of Jenn obtained during the filming of *The Toxic Clouds of 9/11*. Some very moving footage of Jenn appears in my short DVD, *Chemical Sensitivity: A 15-Minute Introduction,* which can be viewed on my website, www.alisonjohnsonmcs.com.

S.C.W.

EPA Attorney

I began working in the Office of Enforcement at the EPA Headquarters in 1984. The EPA was located at the Waterside Mall in southwest Washington, D.C. The privately owned building was designed to be a pair of twelve-story apartment towers connected by a three-story shopping mall.

By the time I moved into my first office in the mall section in 1984, the windows in my office had been permanently bolted shut. Also, the mall area had been divided up into a honeycomb of interior hallways and small private offices surrounding open interior spaces for secretarial and other support staff.

In October 1987, the EPA started installing new carpet in its offices in the Waterside Mall. At that time, I heard about an EPA employee who said that something in her newly renovated office had made her very sick. In fact, she said she had been so sensitized to solvent fumes that she could no longer work in her office. I remember thinking what a sad situation that was and congratulating myself that I was in good health, as usual. Little did I know . . .

In March 1988, I had my first warning that something was seriously unhealthy in my office, but I did not make the connection at the time. The EPA managers were denying that the air quality in the building was bad, and, as I learned later, they were hushing up any incidents like the one I described above. Nevertheless, that March I began to have upper respiratory infections and frequent flu-like symptoms. My doctor would put me on antibiotics and the infection would clear, only to recur a few weeks after I had finished a course of antibiotics. These infections did not keep me away from the office, however; I soldiered on. I wasn't too concerned yet because my health had seemed good prior to the appearance of these respiratory problems. I had previously gone horseback riding three times a week, had jogged three miles several times a week, and had taken aerobics at the EPA Wellness Center.

The first life-threatening crisis I faced was in mid-August of 1988. That morning I left my air-conditioned home and car pooled in an air-conditioned car to the underground garage at the Waterside Mall. After spending about thirty minutes in my air-conditioned office, I began to feel weak and light-headed. I walked over to the EPA Health Unit and almost passed out when I got to the door. I remember the nurse talking to me, shaking me gently, and telling me not to go to sleep. She asked me if I had any chest pains, but I didn't. All I had was a sense of darkness closing in around me and deep fatigue. I remember hearing the nurse tell a doctor that my pulse was 42 and my blood pressure was something just over 50. The next thing I remember is being in an ambulance on the way to the emergency room at George Washington Hospital. Curiously, when I later asked for all the records of my visits to the EPA Health Unit for my lawsuit, there was a conspicuous gap. My August collapse in the building was missing.

The George Washington ER doctor put me on oxygen and released me when my heart rate got up to 50 or so. Strangely enough, the diagnosis on the ER report was "heat exhaustion," despite the fact that I had spent the whole day in air-conditioned places.

When I described what had happened that day during a follow-up visit with a doctor at George Washington Hospital, she assured me that there was nothing wrong with the Waterside Mall. She even suggested that I was unhappy with my job. Even so, she gave me a prescription for oxygen on demand to use at the EPA Health Unit. I became a regular visitor there in the weeks to come. One time when I went in for oxygen, the nurse said they were out. When I asked her how many other EPA employees were coming in for oxygen, she said she was not allowed to give out that information. She advised me to go outside for a while until I felt better.

After my August collapse, my supervisor moved me into another office on the third floor, but this one was located above a first-floor dry cleaning shop. During the time I worked in this office, I often smelled solvents and mold. The number and frequency of my symptoms increased. These symptoms included open sores inside and around my mouth, hoarseness after working in my office for thirty minutes, painful joints, episodes of conjunctivitis with pus running out of my eyes like tears, sensitivity to light so severe that I wore dark glasses in my office with added clip-on dark glasses when I went outside. I also had headaches, upper respiratory infections, and pleurisy, and my skin was so dry that it cracked and bled. I had lost so much hair that I had bald patches on my head that made me look like a chemotherapy patient. My skin had a grey pallor, and I often had painful abdominal spasms. My memory was getting bad, and I noticed that it was taking me longer and longer to collect my thoughts and write assignments. My productivity was declining.

From March through November 1989, I was on antibiotics almost constantly for upper respiratory infections. A few days after I ended a course of treatment, I would develop another infection. I had chronic bronchitis and non-allergic rhinitis. By December 1989, I was taking three antibiotics concurrently without any effect on the upper respiratory infections and pleurisy. My chest and ribs hurt from the hard and almost constant coughing.

My doctor said my immune system was not working, and she wrote a letter to get me out of the Waterside Mall for ten days. My health improved tremendously during the two weeks I spent away from the Waterside Mall.

A few years later I retired from the EPA on work-related disability. The owners of the Waterside Mall building stole my life from me. I lost my health and my career as a government attorney. My husband lost his wife, and my daughter lost her mother.

Because of the chemical injury I sustained while working in the EPA Headquarters in the Waterside Mall, exposure to chemicals in substances like perfume, diesel exhaust, paint, and cleaning products now increases my respiratory problems, headaches, joint pains, and other symptoms.

I sued the Waterside Mall building owners and won (Bahura, et al. v. S.E.W. Investors, et al., D.C. Court of Appeals, 2000). No amount of money can ever compensate me, however, for what my family lost and for the chronic health problems I live with every day.

The disabilities resulting from the Waterside Mall exposures led me to new experiences. I learned how to play piano to regain the use of fine motor skills in my hands. After eighteen years of playing, I am now in third-year piano books, so I am slowly making progress. Therapeutic horseback riding has helped with balance and vertigo. A teacher friend allowed me to be her classroom aide so I could relearn reading and basic math skills to balance my checkbook. Neurofeedback helps with my attention deficit disorder and recurring transient ischemic attacks.

Every day I make an effort to find some joy. Some days it is easier to do than others.

Margaret Ressler

Exxon Valdez Cleanup Worker

I was the assistant to the head of a crew of about thirty people. I was a medic and was also responsible for lunch. It was up to me to organize everything. Every morning we got on the boat and went to some beach. We worked twelve-hour shifts, which was really exhausting. In addition to my other duties, I sprayed steam from a steam gun to try to get the oil of the rocks and off the beaches. You could smell oil everywhere. They gave us yellow rain suits to help keep off the water and oil, but they were cheap, so within minutes you were soaked to the skin. I decided to buy myself a good set of rain gear.

We would try to get down a couple of inches into the sand and gravel with the steam gun so we could move the oil toward the water. They would have an area boomed off and skimmers to pick up the oil and transfer it into a boat. Afterwards we found that the hot water was killing everything on the beaches.

After spending eight weeks on the cleanup, I developed pneumonia and was sent back to Valdez. Some guy met me at the dock and took me to the emergency room. There they told me to go home and rest. When I went back to file for workers' compensation, there were armed guards outside the workers' comp office, which seemed really odd. They were not letting anyone else in. We were told all our medical records had fallen off the boat. I never did get any workers' comp.

I have fibromyalgia and chronic fatigue syndrome now, and I didn't have those before I worked on the spill cleanup. My muscles hurt a lot now, and I can't stand for any length of time. I can't write because I have a palsy in my right hand, and I've had a lot of trouble sleeping since I worked on the oil spill. In July 1990, just a year after I worked on the spill cleanup, my doctor said I was too disabled to work.

I had been a bartender at Eagle River, but I had to quit because I developed chemical sensitivity and reacted to the alcohol fumes, which were pretty strong by the end of the evening. Lots of other chemicals bother me now. I can't use those pine-scented cleaners anymore, and I'm so sensitive to chemicals now that I can't get a perm.

I've heard of three or four people who died after they worked on the spill. One lady was my roommate. We have a meeting every March 27 for Task Force 8, kind of like a reunion. I've gone to a couple and have heard that so and so died.

Before I worked on the oil spill, I was a very active person. I was a hard worker, an original farm girl. I raised three children as a single mom and also raised four foster children. I had a full social life as a bartender, but now that I'm sick I live in a chair and my son takes care of me.

Kelly Colangelo

9/11 Exposure

On September 11, I had just gotten to work at my office in New Jersey when I got an instant message from my sister in California saying a plane had flown into the World Trade Center. All I had to do was turn around and look out the window to see what had happened. The next day I was able to get back into the city, and my brother and I went on a bit of an adventure to get back to our apartments on Johns Street, which is very close to the World Trade Center. Just the amount of dust we encountered walking from Christopher Street in Greenwich Village all the way down to my apartment building was incredible. In China Town we saw dust six inches deep on the sidewalk. I went through a pair of shoes that day.

When I got into my apartment, it looked like it was snowing when I walked in. I had left my windows open, and the dust was about four inches thick on the window sills. Everything was covered in dust–sofa, rugs, toaster oven, coffee maker. I just kind of stood there. I didn't know what to do. Then I heard my brother's voice saying, "There's cops down here and they want you out." I quickly changed my clothes, put a few things in a suitcase, and left.

On the morning of September 14, I had a terrible headache. I was getting a sore throat, and later that day I started having this deep, throaty cough that sounded like I had been a chain smoker for fifteen years. Everybody at work noticed my new cough.

The following weekend I tried to get back to my apartment again. I ended up waiting most of the day on Johns Street with other residents of my building. We stood for hours breathing in that dust that was coming down like snow. They never did let us back into our building to get anything, so I checked into a hotel. That's when the fatigue hit me, just a constant fatigue. I couldn't walk up and down the subway stairs without having shortness of breath. I continued to have coughing fits and an awful headache. I just didn't feel like doing anything. I called in sick for a couple of days and slept and slept. When I also started getting a rash on my face and hands, I began to wonder if all the health problems I had suddenly developed were connected to my 9/11 exposures.

About two weeks later, I found a company to clean my apartment. The man who came to check my apartment sat on the couch and all this dust came out. He said, "Oh, this is the worst one I've seen yet." I said, "You've got to be joking me. I've seen pictures on TV." At any rate, he told me he would get a crew of eight people to come to clean my apartment a week later. In the meantime, I couldn't be in there for more than five or ten minutes without having a hard time breathing. I had to wear a mask the whole time. I would have to go out in the hallway to get some better air, and sometimes I would go down to the lobby and take a breather and then go back up to the trenches.

The day that the cleaners finally came I had to meet them there. All these people just paraded in with some brooms and mops. They were all wearing brand new T-shirts with the cleaning company's name on them. Some guy with a clipboard had probably gathered these people up from around the corner, where they were hanging out on the street in front of Mrs. Field's Cookies. They had rented a dry-type vacuum to clean the upholstery and the rugs, which didn't seem sufficient to me. I did throw out the mattresses from my bed and from my hide-a-bed sofa.

When I moved back into my apartment on September 30, it just smelled awful, like stale dirt. That was because the air outside was still full of dust, like it was snowing, because people hadn't cleaned the tops of buildings or the window sills or the rest of the exterior surfaces of the buildings, so whenever the wind blew the dust was blowing off the buildings. You couldn't open your windows because it would fly right back in. When I turned on the air conditioning unit to get some air circulating, a big burst of grey dust came out. Here my apartment had just been cleaned, and now it was going to get dust all over it again.

I located the filter, which was underneath the HVAC unit, and saw that there was dust four inches thick on it. The company I had hired had obviously not cleaned it. They probably saw it and said, We're not touching it. It's underneath; she'll never look." So I threw the filter away and asked the landlord for another. She told me they were on back order for the whole building. I had to resort to buying cheesecloth and folding it in layers to cover the opening where the air came out of the HVAC unit. I hoped that would catch the larger particles. After a week, that white cheesecloth was black, so until the filters arrived I had to keep changing the cheesecloth to reduce the amount of dust getting back into my apartment.

October came, and people still hadn't cleaned the outside of their buildings. Sometimes I would be walking down the street and when there was a gust of wind, I would have to shield my face because of all that dust blowing off the tops and sides of buildings coming at me again. It was just terrible to be outside. Stores even started putting signs up on their windows that said, "Fresh Air Inside."

The stale smell in my apartment was still awful, and my rash had not gone away yet. Then in the middle of November, I started having gastro-intestinal pains that were so severe that I would writhe in pain in bed. I could barely even pick up the phone to call in sick to work. This acute attack lasted about two days. Finally, when I felt better, I thought at first that it might just have been something that I ate, but I continued to have substantial GI symptoms, which made food poisoning seem unlikely.

Then December came, and my various symptoms were still there. Nothing had gotten better, so I went to my doctor and told him what had been happening. I said, "Could this have anything to do with what I'm living in?" He replied, "I doubt it. Maybe you should see a psycho-logist." I changed doctors after that appointment. I wasn't ever going back to that one.

I decided that at the beginning of January, I would make a decision about whether to move out of my apartment, which still smelled bad. In early January, when I heard that the WTC fires were at last out, I opened my windows one night, one, two three, and what came out? All the dust out of the window frames blew right into my apartment. It was all over the floor again, all over my sofa again, and on the window sill. I sent it away for testing, and they detected asbestos in four of the five samples that I sent. I still had three months on my lease, but I said, "You know what? My life is more important than my lease."

I moved to midtown, and within a week I felt so much better. The cough was still there, but the sore throats disappeared and the fatigue got better. I still had some gastrointestinal problems, but the headaches had stopped. That was such a big event for me because it had been so difficult to go to work every day with a pounding headache.

After I had been in midtown for about eight months, I decided to move back to Lower Manhattan because I missed my old neighborhood. I succeeded in finding an apartment building in the WTC area that had been thoroughly cleaned and seemed free of the WTC dust. I feel so much better now and have been able to get over some of the terrible symptoms that I had after 9/11.

Although my general health is much improved, a few years after 9/11 I noticed that I was becoming very sensitive to certain smells like perfumes, colognes, cigarette smoke, and diesel fuel. When I walk down the sidewalk and somebody is smoking, I could just scream. I just can't stand the smell anymore. When someone is wearing too much cologne, I have to get away from them. I hold my breath now when I walk by buses because the diesel smell is too much for me to handle and gives me a headache. This chemical sensitivity may be a troublesome legacy from all the toxic dust I breathed after 9/11.

Mark

Former Videomaker

It's Christmas morning in the Northwest. And, for the eleventh Christmas in a row, I am sitting in my car, hanging out in a city park, trying to stay warm and dry. I'm forty-nine years old and have multiple chemical sensitivity (MCS). Like many others with MCS, I also suffer from chronic fatigue immune dysfunction syndrome (CFIDS). My MCS is severe enough that for the past eleven years I've been unable to go inside a house or building for any length of time before I start reacting to something. Severe enough that I've been forced to live in my twenty-two-year old car, which lost long ago that "new car smell."

What I react to depends on the situation. Sometimes it's the personal care products people are wearing, like perfumes, deodorants, lotions, and hair spray. Sometimes it's the carpets, computers, furniture, and plastics in a room that are "off-gassing" chemical compounds. Sometimes I react to pesticides, cleaning products, or the chemicals off-gassing from paint. Indoor air is a heavily polluted soup of chemical compounds to which my body reacts adversely.

My reactions vary depending on the type of chemical pollutant I'm exposed to. My most frequent reactions are blinding headaches, a nasty metallic taste, tingly face, hoarseness, difficulty breathing, burning lungs, and stinging eyes. Less frequent but much more serious reactions are throat closure, asthma, chest pains, dizziness, and disorientation.

So in my old out-gassed car I am sitting in a park on Christmas morning; the park for the time being is "safe" (meaning I'm not reacting to anything). However, this could change at any moment because outdoor air is heavily polluted as well. In some areas, various types of industry, big or small, are belching out chemical pollutants. Many homes are polluting the surrounding air by burning wood or synthetic logs. Every house has a dryer vent, and the smell of detergent and the fabric softener in dryer sheets can travel a considerable distance. What also drifts, especially with a breeze, are the fertilizers, pesticides, and herbicides that are used around homes and other buildings. Local and state governments are heavy users of these products, especially herbicides. The roadsides people walk and bike on are regularly sprayed to keep noxious weeds from growing. Living in my car, I spend a good deal of time in the parks in my area; these are also sprayed and fertilized at various times of the year. And of course the exhaust from cars, trucks, and buses is a large source of pollution.

As you can see, living in my car and spending most of my time outside is not a good solution to my problem. On a daily basis I have to pick or guess which will be better or worse, indoor pollution or outdoor pollution. For me, the more tolerable environment is usually outdoors. The simple fact is I'm mobile, and when a problem suddenly arises in one area, I can move to a different area away from the offending chemical pollutants. The challenge, of course, is in trying to out-maneuver or outrun the pervasiveness of chemical pollutants in the air.

I'm often reacting and therefore frequently moving. I drive 2,000 to 3,000 miles per month; much of that mileage is the result of moving around to try to find a safe spot. The bottom line is that I spend almost all my time in my car, exhausted, sick, in pain, and always on the move.

Genetic Predisposition

I became ill and disabled with chronic fatigue immune dysfunction syndrome (CFIDS) shortly after my thirty-fifth birthday. Approximately two years later, at the age of thirty-seven, I developed multiple chemical sensitivity (MCS). When I called to inform my family of my new MCS symptoms, they reminded me that I had been "sensitive" all my life. This shocked me. I never thought of myself as being "sensitive" and didn't think anyone else saw me that way either. However, reflecting back I quickly realized this had all started when I was a child.

There I was six or seven years old, sitting in the back seat of a car with my brother and sister. My mom was sitting up front in the passenger seat, and one of her girlfriends was driving. It was wintertime and frigid in upstate New York. The windows were rolled up, and my mom and her friend were smoking cigarettes and gabbing as we drove along. The inside of the windows were fogged up, and the smoke in the car was so thick I could barely see. I was choking on the smoke and gasping for air. I felt like I was suffocating, so I pulled the collar of my shirt up over my nose to filter out the smoke. When my mom saw what

I was doing, she scoffed and yelled at me, "Oh Mark, it's not that bad!" She and her friend then cracked their windows ever so slightly and continued to smoke and gab away.

When I was growing up, I spent many hours alone in my bedroom, angry that I couldn't be in the living room to watch TV with the rest of my family because my mom was chain smoking. In my late teens, my buddies and I would hit the bars and taverns for a good time (drinking age was eighteen back then). Predictably, I was greeted by a thick blanket of cigarette smoke in these places. My burning eyes and lungs would force me to go outside every twenty minutes or so, in all types of weather, to get some fresh air.

Then there was the "beehive" hairdo of that time. As she was getting ready to go out, my mom would spray half a can of hair spray on her mountainous hairdo. Much of the house would fill with this visible cloud of hair spray that made me choke. My mom would come out of the bathroom all smiles and ask us kids how she looked. While trying to hold my breath, I'd mutter that she looked good and then would quickly run to my bedroom so I could breathe.

It wasn't until my early twenties that I started having problems with perfume. This became evident because my girlfriend at the time was always trying out some new brand of perfume. I found the scent of a couple of them to be pleasing and had no trouble tolerating those ones, but the others would give me pounding headaches.

Looking back on the first thirty-plus years of my life, I remember being generally healthy. All through my school years, I was an athlete. In high school, I earned ten letters in football and track. During my twenties, I became an avid backpacker, rock climber, and mountaineer. I was well educated, earning a B.S. in Telecommunications with a graduate-level minor in Instructional Technology. I was well grounded, had a good social life with several close friends, and had a healthy love life. After finishing college, I was making a living in the video production industry, working on corporate/instructional videos and selling professional video equipment.

My high level of good health was confirmed when I went to a cardiologist for a full workup at the age of thirty. The cardiologist said that my treadmill results were better "than most high school basketball players that run up and down the court all day."

At the age of thirty-one, I joined a small exclusive athletic club that catered to marathon runners, triathletes, competitive cyclists, etc. Since I was a new member, the trainer did a complete workup on me that included a cardiopulmonary test. The tests he did indicated that I had the cardiopulmonary capacity of an Olympic athlete.

Thus at age thirty-two, I was very healthy. I was also happy and a highly motivated person. Cigarette smoke, hair sprays, and perfumes were an inconvenience (a.k.a. pain in the ass), but I dealt with them. I never thought of them as an indicator of me being "sensitive" or as a precursor of things to come.

The Day I Broke

Then something happened, though I'm not sure what, and I began to develop an array of health problems. Though I was slowly coming to the realization that something was starting to go wrong with me, I still had plenty of energy and had no interest in seeing doctors. So for the next two to three years, I endured an ever-increasing amount of physical symptoms. I herniated a disc in my lower back, tore both rotator cuffs in my shoulders, tore my right knee cartilage, and developed advanced degenerative arthritis in my left knee (a by-product of a football knee surgery). I also developed persistent pain in my neck, elbow, and hip. I was having severe memory problems, sleep problems, and libido problems. If that wasn't enough, I also developed G.I. symptoms– constipation, bloating, cramping, and heartburn. In addition, I developed heart palpitations and chronic prostatitis (infection of the prostate). I was freezing year round with cold extremities. I became hypoglycemic (low blood sugar) and sensitive to sounds like music, kids playing, lawnmowers, and people talking. And, finally, not a month or two would pass that I was not fighting off a cold or flu.

Then came the day I crossed the line. I remember "the day I broke" vividly–I was thirty-five, and one afternoon I was sitting in a Lazy Boy chair napping. When I woke up, I quickly realized something was wrong. I had no energy, none! Eventually, I got the strength to get up from the chair, but within a couple of hours I was developing classic flu-like symptoms. Although I stayed home from work most of the next week, sick enough to stay in bed, I was getting worse with each passing day. When I finally dragged myself to the doctor's office, I was diagnosed with an inner ear infection, strep throat, bronchitis, a swollen liver, and mononucleosis. I was given antibiotics and instructions of bed rest and no work for the next three or four weeks.

While I was lying in bed during those weeks, sicker than I'd ever been in my life, one of my roommates, who was a landscaper, decided to put in a brand new lawn, complete with fertilizer and herbicides. He also sprayed the many bushes that surrounded the house with pesticides and sprinkled around the garbage cans some pellets of a pesticide that is now banned. I could smell the pesticide and fertilizer as I lay in bed trying to recuperate. It was ten miserable, bed-ridden weeks later before I was able to muster the energy to return to work on a part-time basis. I was better, but far from well.

During my sick leave, the company I worked for had relocated its offices to a different building. Everything in this office space was new–carpet, paint, desks, furniture, computers, etc. We were all excited about the move to the new space, but my return to work lasted only one week. I awoke one night with severe heart palpitations that sent me to the emergency room and put me into a severe relapse. I was subsequently laid off by my company and haven't worked since. This was the start of my journey through the medical establishment maze. I saw doctor after doctor who had no idea what was wrong with me. This didn't stop them from writing a prescription–usually for anti-depressants or anti-anxiety drugs. Thinking that the doctors knew best, I would take whatever they prescribed, only to have some type of an adverse reaction. Again the doctors were perplexed.

It wasn't until six months after "the day I broke" that I went to a doctor who was a pain specialist and was given the diagnosis of chronic fatigue immune dysfunction syndrome (CFIDS). He explained that people with CFIDS are more sensitive to prescription drugs and need to start with smaller doses. For well over a year and a half, I worked with this doctor, diligently taking my medications and adhering to his advice, but there was no improvement. I wasn't getting better; I was getting worse. I was still in a chronic state of exhaustion and continued to have flu-like symptoms, with new symptoms appearing almost daily. I was barely able to function, and I was miserable.

Making the Connection

One of those new symptoms was the increase in my sense of smell. I don't remember the trigger. All I know is that suddenly I could smell. I mean really smell. I had lived in the same house, with the same roommates, for five and a half years with no problems in the past. Now I was complaining to my roommates on a daily basis about the smell of the laundry soap, the painting done in the garage, the mothballs in my roommate's closet, the cleaners and bleaches.

The connection came after a couple of weeks of dealing with my new symptoms. A friend called who thought it would be good for me to get out of the house and go to a matinee. She offered to drive because she wanted to show off her brand-new Toyota Celica. It was a beautiful summer day, and the windows were down as we drove to the theater. The drive was only fifteen minutes, but by the time we arrived I wasn't feeling good at all. I stood outside the theater for a moment trying to decide if we should go ahead with the movie or if I should have my friend take me back home. Since I had been feeling fine just fifteen minutes earlier, I thought I must have eaten something for lunch that was bothering me. I was well aware of food sensitivities at this stage and had tested positive for several foods.

I finally decided to go in, and by the time the movie started I was feeling better. After the movie, we jumped back in her new car and headed home. Five minutes into the drive I started feeling awful again. It was another ten minutes before we got to my place, and by then I was in trouble. I was having difficulty talking, swallowing, and breathing. My throat was closing up. My friend was concerned and asked if she should take me to the emergency room. I said no and instinctively jumped out of the car to get some fresh air. Within a couple of minutes, my symptoms began to clear and I started to wonder about what had happened that afternoon. Why was I OK before she picked me up, but then felt awful after the short drive to the theater? Why did I feel better during the movie? And why, after another short drive in my friend's new car, am I practically 9-1-1 material? That's when it struck me like a bolt of lightening. It's the smell of the new car! It's the smell of the off-gassing chemicals in the new car! It's the chemicals from my roommates' pesticides, laundry soap, paints, mothballs, cleaners, and bleaches that have been making me sick! Holy Shit, I'm chemically sensitive!

Increasing Levels of MCS

I was thirty-seven years old when I had the revelation that I was chemically sensitive. I'm now forty-nine, and looking back, I can clearly see that the severity of my affliction progressed through several distinct levels, each one building on the other.

At first, when I would smell an offending chemical odor (perfume, paint, detergents, etc.), I would have an adverse physical reaction (headaches, breathing difficulties, metallic taste, dizziness, etc.). When I left that environment, my reactions would clear. Unfortunately, my list was growing with incredible speed. Every day I was discovering something new I was reacting to. It was this "spreading phenomenon" that made it intolerable for me to live in the same house with the same roommates I had lived with for the past five and a half years. Life there became a daily bombardment of chemical smells that produced in me terrible physical reactions. My attempts to seal myself in my bedroom by closing the door, heater vent, and windows didn't work. It was a losing battle; the chemical smells still got in. Not to mention that I still needed to use the bathroom and the kitchen. I soon realized that I would have to move out.

I got lucky though (or so I thought), and through a friend I met a lady with fibromyalgia who said she was committed to helping me get better. However, after just one month of continual exposures to her pesticides, fertilizers, nail polish, and daily guests wearing colognes and perfumes, I was once again looking for a place to live. For the next two years, this scenario was repeated over and over. During this time, while still in a state of extreme illness, I made over two thousand phone calls to ask about rooms for rent and I moved sixteen times. I was bouncing around never knowing from day to day where I might be spending the night.

I spent two weeks in a friend's moldy trailer with the windows wide open during the middle of winter. Another two weeks on a friend's couch and another week on a friend's basement floor. I spent three months in a shared living situation with five others who all claimed to understand MCS. Nevertheless, I remember going to bed several nights fully clothed in my winter gear–down jacket and wool hat–with the windows wide open because my roommates were painting their rooms or using hair coloring solutions or colognes and perfumes. I even spent several winter months in my tent, constantly setting it up and taking it down as I bounced from one friend's backyard to another. For about eight months, I lived in a house with gas fumes that came from a leak in a downstairs apartment with a faulty range. The landlord finally called the gas company because of my nonstop complaining, and the gas company found a significant leak. When she was forced to buy a new range, she was furious at me.

I was in a downward spiral, and the crux of my problem was my ever-increasing chemical sensitivities. Just when I thought the situation couldn't get any worse, once again my chemical sensitivities progressed to a new level. I was now starting to react to odors that had been absorbed by my hair or my clothes. If I shook hands, hugged, or even stood next to someone wearing perfume or cologne, invariably my clothes and hair would absorb some of the fragrance that I would then react to. This scenario was occurring daily, and it wasn't just to perfumes and colognes. If I went into a building or a room that had been recently painted, I would come away smelling of paint. Or maybe the floors had just been washed and waxed or the carpet had been shampooed. Again, I'd come away smelling of these chemicals. Cigarette smoke is a classic example that most non-smokers are well aware of–that nasty smell gets on everything. And let's not forget the fun task of going to a gas station, where small puddles of gasoline are everywhere and gasoline vapors saturate the air.

To minimize my exposure to these odors, I stopped shaking hands and hugging people and started hurrying in and out of buildings and stores. But I soon realized that no matter how quick I was, if there was an odor in the air enough of it would cling to my hair and clothes to cause a reaction in me. The number one offender was the widespread use of air fresheners and deodorizers. It seemed that no matter where I went I was being exposed to these products–in homes, cars, malls, libraries, grocery stores, public bathrooms, and even in some health food stores. On a daily basis, I was getting odors on my clothes and in my hair that would cause me to react until I was able to shower and launder my clothes.

The endless ordeal of having to gather the strength to move sixteen times over this two-year period, when I was constantly feeling so sick, had brought me to the breaking point. The situation had become so intolerable that I had to make some serious changes in my lifestyle. I had to rethink how and where I could live. The solution to "how" was simple–avoidance. I felt I had no choice but to avoid going into most homes and buildings as well as to drastically reduce my contact with people. As for the solution to "where" I was going to live, this was a more complicated matter. I was now living on a small monthly check from Social Security Disability Income. This meant that I could not afford to live alone so that I could control my environment but would instead have to opt for a shared living situation with several other people. But I had already gone this route and found it to be an exercise in futility because it was impossible for me to control the various products that roommates would want to use. Simply put, there was only one option left; enter my new home–a 1981 VW Vanagon. I threw my futon in the back of the van and felt this was going to be the beginning of my road to recovery. Unfortunately, this new life style came with a whole new world of unforeseen challenges.

Long Nights

To start with, where should I sleep? Or rather, where should I park so that I can sleep in my vehicle? Trying to find a place to park and sleep turned out to be a juggling act. I quickly learned that most people don't like the idea of someone sleeping in their vehicle, especially in their neighborhood. I try to avoid anyone noticing me by waiting until 11 P.M. to go to bed. By that hour, I figure most people are done walking their dogs, cats, ferrets, and armadillos and have settled in for the night. I keep my vehicle clean, and I also work hard to keep up my physical appearance so I won't be viewed as a menace or a street person. Regardless, I still have had the police knock on my vehicle window more times than I can remember. Startled from my sleep, disoriented and blinded by their high beams, spotlights, and flashlights, I can feel my heart pounding. Yes, officer; no, officer. I live in my vehicle, officer. No, I haven't been drinking; no, I have no weapons. All the time I'm hoping they don't want me to get out of my car and do a sobriety test. With my CFIDS, low blood pressure problems, dizzy spells, and loss of coordination, I just might fail. I also hope they won't want to search my vehicle. Everything I own is in my vehicle. I wouldn't be able to handle the stress of them going through everything, nor find the energy to put it back.

I have to balance these encounters with the police with the encounters I have with partying teenagers. I've lost a lot of sleep on the many occasions when a car-load of teenagers has pulled in and parked right next to me. The teenagers I run into in the middle of the night are usually fearless, defiant, and high. They don't care how much noise they're making as they crank up their car stereos, bust bottles, throw trash around, and even vandalize property. My heart is always in my throat pounding away when this happens. Are these kids harmless or are they feeling destructive? Have they noticed my vehicle, can they see me inside? Maybe it's all cool and I should just ride it out, or maybe I shouldn't wait to find out and should leave.

Despite the fact that I park in the nice areas of town, I've had to deal with this situation dozens and dozens and dozens of times. I've had the pleasure of being awakened by youths attempting to pour beer down my gas tank. I've woken up when my car started violently rocking because some kids thought it would be fun to jump up and down on my trunk. I've been awakened by the sound of my rear window being smashed as a youth attempted to steal my belongings in the rear seat. And on several occasions, I've been awakened by the unmistakable sounds of two youths "doing it." Say what you will, but when these events happen (usually between 1 and 4 A.M.), I can't help but wonder about their parents.

Let's now add a third component to my nightly juggling act. The real challenge is to find a place to park and sleep that is MCS safe. It is a challenge to which I have no solution and one that I battle with every night. Simply put, there are no safe places for me to sleep, and the situation changes from night to night. What worked for me last night might not work for me tonight, and vice versa.

My nightly ritual begins at 11 P.M. when I pull up to a spot, stick my head out of the window, and start sniffing like a dog. Half the time I can't smell anything; the other half I can. What I usually smell is fabric softener and laundry soap coming from dryer vents and smoke coming from chimneys. I can smell pesticides, herbicides, and fertilizers if they have been applied within the last week. Depending on the wind direction, I can smell emissions from local industries. Many times I smell some type of chemical substance but cannot identify it. Either way, whenever I smell something problematic, I start my vehicle and am on the move. I drive to a different spot and repeat the procedure.

I keep moving, repeating this procedure until I find a spot where I'm not detecting any chemical odors. Once I find such a place I lie down to get some badly needed sleep. But wait, now my head is pounding or my face is tingling. Maybe my eyes are burning, or I'm getting a nasty metallic taste in my mouth. But I didn't smell anything, so I tell myself, "I'm not moving; I'm too tired, mind over matter!" But all my reactions are becoming more severe and intolerable. So I get up, stick my head back out the window to double check. Sniff, sniff; nope, no smell. Yet my head feels like it is going to explode with pain. In a state of fatigued rage, I start my vehicle and move on. Within minutes, my reactions clear.

I realize when I start my night that it's a 50/50 shot that the first place I hit will work for me. On a bad night, I can spend hours moving from one spot to another. I've moved as many as fifteen times in one night (a Guinness Book record). My body, mind, and psyche are usually fried by this point. To complicate the situation even more, just as I have to go to bed late in order not to be spotted, I have to get up at 6 A.M.for the same reason.

I had lived in my van for two years when one fateful day, while I was inside taking a shower at the local pool, someone plowed into my parked van. The van was totaled, and now I was really homeless. I was rescued by some good friends, and needing something quick I purchased a 1986 Oldsmobile car. Instead of a comfortable futon in the back, I now had a cramped split bench seat in the front that I used, and continue to use today, as a bed. Good times.

A Day in a Life

After struggling through the night to find a place to park my car and sleep–it was a great night, four hours of tossing and turning–I'm now up at 6 A.M. I can quickly tell what kind of a day it will be. Either I'll be a zombie–sick and exhausted all day–or I'll feel halfway decent and will want to take on the world. In the latter case, I'll have my best energy and clearest mind in the morning, so that's when I do whatever it is I have to do. I hit one of the health food stores to pick up my breakfast. Because I do not have the ability to store, wash, prepare, or cook food, all my food comes from the deli counter. Certainly easy, but rather expensive and very boring. Also, it makes it difficult to stay away from the foods I may be allergic to. Four times a week, I'll take a shower at the YMCA or at one of the local public pools after I have had breakfast. This is a problem not only because of the chlorine vapors, from the pool and jacuzzi, but also because of the dozens of personal care products that are used in locker rooms. Despite taking the world's fastest showers (another Guinness Book record), I'm still gasping for fresh air when I leave these facilities.

As needed, usually twice a week, I pick up my mail at a local UPS store where I have a box. Until recently this has never posed a problem, but my sensitivity has increased so much that I am now unable to enter the store at all. Luckily, the owner and employees have come to know me and understand my situation. They now run my mail outside to me when they see me drive up. I'm extremely grateful, but always feel a twinge of embarrassment when they hand me my mail.

Until a few years ago, I was able to wash my clothes at a laundromat, albeit it was a very tricky ordeal. To minimize my exposures, I would arrive at the laundromat as soon as the doors opened at 6 or 7 A.M., long before others arrived with their detergents and bleaches. I'd run an empty washer and dryer through their cycles a couple of times before I'd add my clothes. This helped get rid of the detergent or dryer sheet residue in the machines. I would then do a load of laundry using an all-natural detergent.

Unfortunately, I am now so sensitive that I can no longer use a laundromat, so the UPS store has become my laundry drop. Once a month one of the UPS store employees will meet me outside, and I will hand them one or two bags containing my dirty laundry. They then take the bags into the store, box them up, and send them to my brother in Texas, who is my "clothes man." When my dirty laundry arrives, he runs an empty washing machine through a couple of rinse cycles to wash away any detergent residue. Then he washes my soiled clothes with a natural soap, rinses them a few times, and dries them before returning them to me. He also purchases all my new clothes and washes them many times to get out the chemicals used in the fabric finishes.

OK, back to my day. I've eaten, showered, and picked up my mail. Next I'll make a few phone calls on my cell phone, and afterwards it's time to attend to other business. Occasionally, I have an appointment with a doctor or dentist. Or some days I end up at my mechanics' shop. I upgraded my car from an '86 Olds to an '87 Olds that is clocking in with over 290,000 miles. My car is really–and unfortunately–my life. Much of my time revolves around keeping it clean, organized, and operating properly. Driving my car an average of 2,000 to 3,000 miles a month tends to cause a lot of wear and tear, so costly repairs are not infrequent. Having my car worked on is always a stressful experience. Auto repair shops are extremely toxic environments for me, and I don't have the luxury of dropping my car off or even relaxing in the waiting room. I have to wait outside the shop the entire time. Surprise! My car never seems to need major maintenance or repairs during the nice summer weather. But again, I'm lucky in that my mechanics know me and my story very well. They bend over backwards to accommodate me and to minimize exposures to me and my car's interior.

Mornings are also a time when I do any paperwork I may have, which is another big challenge. I commonly react to paper and the inks used, and if someone else has handled the paperwork prior to my getting it, it might have cologne, perfume, or cigarette odors clinging to it. Finally, I'll often take this time of the day to straighten up and organize my car. But it's approaching lunch-time, so it's off to the deli department at my nearby health food store.

After lunch I start to fade fast and pretty much become non-functional. I need to find a park that I can tolerate to crash in for the afternoon. It's now nap time, that is, if it's spring or fall. It can be difficult to fall asleep in the summer when the temperature in my car easily hits one hundred degrees. Who needs a sauna when I get a good sweat right in my car? Winters in the Northwest bring non-stop rains, and the temperature inside my car drops down into the very damp and chilly forties. In nice weather, parks can be quite noisy from people driving through, car doors slamming shut, dogs barking, and kids playing. Then there's America's youth, who have to announce to the world that they've arrived with their screams and cranked-up car stereo systems. Even though it's a struggle, I usually recline my seat and manage to take a light nap for an hour or so.

Though my body badly needed a nap, when I awake I'm anything but refreshed. I'm totally exhausted, and it takes a while before I'm even able to stand because of my low blood pressure. After I pull out of my brain-fog funk, I get my supplements ready and prepare my daytimer for another big day tomorrow. I check my phone messages and do some light stretching outside my car. The truth of the matter is that I'm just killing time until dinner. I'd like to tell you that I have big plans for dinner tonight. Yeah, I'm going out on a hot date to a nice restaurant. But instead I'll be eating my third pre-made sandwich of the day.

After dinner time, I get what might be considered a second wind. Often I attempt to go to various libraries (public, university) to do some research on MCS and CFIDS via the Internet and books. Having knowledge about my condition is invaluable when I'm working with doctors. Not only is my office visit more efficient, but it also helps me determine which doctors really know what they're talking about and which ones are a waste of time.

Try as I might to get into these libraries, it is extremely challenging because of the many exposures from everyone's scented personal-care products. Instead, most evenings I end up at one of my safe parks and just hang out in my car, thinking in the dark for hours. I'd like to tell you that I'm relaxed and meditating, but I'm too busy looking over my shoulder for those pesky partying teenagers, creeps, and the cops. I don't listen to the radio. Being sound sensitive, I can't handle the FM music stations, plus I'm not much of a fan of what's played on commercial radio. When it comes to the AM talk-radio stations, I'll pass on those too. My nervous system can't handle the hate-filled tone of these stations. Rather, I just sit and think about how this all happened to me. How did it start, and, most importantly, how do I fix it? I also fantasize about a world in which it's common sense for people not to smoke, use pesticides, cologne, or air fresheners. I fantasize about a time when people will truly understand. A time when people will look back and wonder, "What the hell were we thinking?" I think about these things a lot. Until finally it's 11 P.M., and once again I'll start my search for a safe place to park and sleep.

The absolute worst thing about being part of this mad experiment gone awry is that I have no social life. Put simply, this disorder is very isolating. I'm alone and mind-numbingly bored all the time. About the only interaction I have is with the cashiers I see daily at the health food store, the receptionists at my doctors/dentists, and of course my mechanics. Maybe once or twice during the summer I'll meet up with a friend at a park.

As for my family, they are extremely supportive of me and my situation, though it's been a long time since I've seen my brother and sister because they live in distant states. My mom died of breast cancer a couple of years ago in New York. Unfortunately, I couldn't travel that far to see her at the end or even go to her funeral service. When my father and stepmother retired, they moved to a city only a five-hour drive away. The drive is difficult for me, but I've been able to do it a couple of times. However, I'm unable to stay long at their place because I usually end up reacting to all the yard work or remodeling that their neighbors are always doing. Luckily, there is a state park close by where I can hang out until I head back to my home turf.

Tip of the Iceberg

The other night while I was sitting in my car in one of the parks I frequent, a police officer drove in and approached my car. He was not in a good mood and angrily told me that the park was closed and then asked what I was doing. I politely corrected him and said that the park was indeed still open for several more hours. This only pissed him off even more, so he grabbed his 9mm pistol out of his holster. Holding his pistol in one hand and a flashlight in the other, the officer noticed my bags of clothes and blankets in the rear seat. He snapped at me, "It looks like you have a body back there" and demanded to know what the contents were. I quickly reached back and lifted my blanket and opened several of my bags to show him there was no threat. I was trying to calm him down as I handed him my ID.

After running a check on me, he came back to my car a little calmer and started to ask me questions about why I was living in my car. I politely explained to him my health issues and said that I was very allergic to chemicals. In response, the police officer growled out, "You're a real mess." He continued to comment about me being in the park at night all alone, about my clothes in bags, and about me being Mr. Allergic. He finished by saying that he had been on the force for twenty years and that this was "the weirdest damn thing" he had ever seen. I nodded my head in agreement and thought to myself, if he only knew the whole story.

The whole story is that I've been disabled and ill for fifteen years, during eleven of which I've been homeless and living in my vehicle because of my sensitivities to practically everything. And as you might imagine, I have quite a collection of unusual stories. These last few pages have been a mere introduction; the whole story would take volumes.

What's interesting is that once people learn even a little bit about my story, their usual response is, "How do you do it?" Or better yet, they ask, "What keeps you going?" I usually just shrug my shoulders to indicate, "Hell if I know!" But one thing I do know is that if it were not for the support of my family, I would not have made it this long. Unlike so many others with MCS that I've met, whose families have abandoned them, mine hasn't. And though my brother and sister live across the country, they understand my condition and continue to believe in me and help out when they can, just as my dad and stepmother do. I realize how difficult it sometimes is on them; they have families and overly full schedules of their own, yet they are always there for me.

Over the past fifteen years of my illness, I've had a few good friends. They've been the ones on the front lines with me, listening to my wild rants, the daily horror stories. (Fortunately, I fairly quickly realized that there was a limit to how much of this stuff I could burden my friends with. At that point, I bought a mini tape recorder, and each night I would sit in my car and vent into the recorder. It probably saved my sanity and my friendships.) On numerous occasions, my friends have literally saved my ass (i.e., my van was totaled in an auto accident, and my car has broken down way too many times). Though many of them have moved on and I haven't seen them in years, I will forever be grateful for the tremendous help they were to me when I needed them.

I also happen to be very philosophical about life and have plenty of time to reflect on my illness. It gives me a sense of purpose at this point. I can't change the world, but I can plant a little seed of information about multiple chemical sensitivity with everyone I meet. More and more people are becoming familiar with MCS, and the day will come when everyone will know about this condition and understand it. I like to think of myself as a modern-day Johnny Appleseed.

The bottom line is I know many other people who have it worse in life. I see them daily–the truly homeless who have nobody to help them out, the blind with their walking sticks, the handicapped who putter around busy streets in their breath-controlled, motorized wheelchairs. And the elderly who sit alone, looking out the windows of their homes, wishing they could be outside walking or driving a car like me. And finally, the extremely ill of all ages who are bedridden and in need of constant medical attention until the day they die. I'm lucky compared to them. I still have a passion for life and honestly believe that one day I'll, once again, be able to put it to use.

Editor's Note: Because of Mark's health problems and his limited access to computers, he first wrote this story in longhand in his car. It was then typed up by his sister, heavily edited by his brother, and further edited by me.

The trials of Job would be an apt description for the last fifteen years of Mark's life. I have met with him several times on a couple of trips to his city and found him a very likeable person. We talk occasionally by phone. I am impressed by the mental balance and tremendous courage Mark has maintained under circumstances so difficult that most people would have given up by now.

Note to the Reader

For further information about multiple chemical sensitivity, the reader may wish to visit the website of the Chemical Sensitivity Foundation, www.chemicalsensitivityfoundation.org. One of the Foundation's main goals is to raise public awareness about chemical sensitivity, and it will be giving a copy of this book to every member of Congress in early 2009. Funds permitting, we will also give copies to other government officials, reporters, physicians in positions of influence, and many others who help shape public opinion.

On my personal website, www.alisonjohnsonmcs.com, various excerpts from my four documentaries can be played. These include some of the people whose stories appear in Part II.

There are many important topics that are not covered in the present book. Many chemically sensitive readers will want more information about reducing toxic exposures in their home, handling the new food intolerances faced by so many people with MCS, interfacing effectively with the medical and disability systems, and dealing with disbelief. For these readers, I wish to recommend the following book by a faculty member of James Madison University who serves on the board of the Chemical Sensitivity Foundation:

Multiple Chemical Sensitivity
A Survival Guide

by Pamela Reed Gibson

www.earthrivebooks.com

Selected Bibliography of Studies
on Chemical Sensitivity
in Peer-Reviewed Journals
2008 Version

Antelman, S.M. "Time-Dependent Sensitization in Animals: A Possible Model of Multiple Chemical Sensitivity in Humans." *Toxicology and Industrial Health* 10, nos. 4-5 (July-October 1994*)*: 335-42.

Arnold Liamosas, P.A., Arrizabalaga Clement, P., Bonet Agusti, M., de la Fuente Brull, X. "Multiple Chemical Sensitivity in Sick-Building Syndrome.*" Medicina Clinica (Barcelona)* 126, no. 20 (May 27, 2006): 774-78.

Association of Occupational and Environmental Clinics. "Advancing the Understanding of Multiple Chemical Sensitivity." *Toxicology and Industrial Health* 8, no. 4 (1992): 1.

Ashford, N., Heinzow, B., Lütjen, K., Marouli, C., Mølhave, L, Mönch, B., Papadopoulos, S., Rest, K., Rosdahl, D., Siskos, P., Velonakis, E., et al. "Chemical Sensitivity in Selected European Countries: An Exploratory Study." A Report to the European Commission. *Ergonomia*, 1995. Athens, Greece.

ATSDR (Agency for Toxic Substances and Disease Registry). "Proceedings of the Conference on Low-Level Exposure to Chemicals and Neurobiologic Sensitivity." *Toxicology and Industrial Health* 10, nos. 4-5 (1994): 25.

Baines, C.J., McKeown-Eyssen, G.E., Riley, N., Cole, D.E., Marshall, L., Loescher, B., Jazmaji, V. "Case-Control Study of Multiple Chemical Sensitivity, Comparing Haematology, Biochemistry, Vitamins and Serum Volatile Organic Compound Measures." *Occupational Medicine* 54, no. 6 (September 2004): 408-18.

Bartha, L., Baumzweiger, W., Buscher, D., Callender, M., Dahl, K., Davidoff, A., et al. "Multiple Chemical Sensitivity: A 1999 Consensus." *Archives of Environmental Health* 54, no. 3 (1999): 147-49.

Bascom, R. "Multiple Chemical Sensitivity: A Respiratory Disorder." *Toxicology and Industrial Health* 8, no. 4 (1991): 221-28.

Bascom, R., Meggs, W., Frampton, M., Hudnell, K., Killburn, K., Kobal, G., Medinsky, M., and Rea, W. "Neurogenic Inflammation: With Additional Discussion of Central and Perceptual Integration of Nonneurogenic Inflammation." *Environmental Health Perspectives* 105, Supplement 2 (1997): 531-37.

Bell, I. R. "Clinically Relevant EEG Studies and Psychophysiological Findings: Possible Neural Mechanisms for Multiple Chemical Sensitivity." *Toxicology* 111 (1996): 101-17.

Bell, I.R. "White Paper: Neuropsychiatric Aspects of Sensitivity to Low-Level Chemicals: A Neural Sensitization Model." *Toxicology and Industrial Health* 10, nos. 4-5 (July-October 1994): 277-312.

Bell, I., Baldwin, C.M., Schwartz, G.E. "Sensitization Studies in Chemically Intolerant Individuals: Implications for Individual Difference Research." *Annals of the New York Academy of Science* 453 (2001): 38-47.

Bell, I., Baldwin, C., Fernandez, M., and Schwartz, G. "Neural Sensitization Model for Multiple Chemical Sensitivity: Overview of Theory and Empirical Evidence." *Toxicology and Industrial Health* 15, nos. 3-4 (1999): 295-304.

Bell, I., Rossi, J., Gilbert, M., Kobal, G., Morrow, L., Newlin, D., Sorg, B., and Wood, R. "Testing the Neural Sensitization and Kindling Hypothesis for Illness from Low Levels of Environmental Chemicals." *Environmental Health Perspectives* 105, Supplement 2 (1997): 539-47.

Berg, N.D., Linneberg, A., Dirksen, A., Elberling, J. "Phenotypes of Individuals Affected by Airborne Chemicals in the General Population." *International Archives of Occupational and Environmental Health* (August 28, 2008).

Berg, N.D., Linneberg, A., Dirksen, A., Elberling, J. "Prevalence of Self-Reported Symptoms and Consequences Related to Inhalation of Airborne Chemicals in a Danish General Population." *International Archives of Occupational and Environmental Health* 81, no. 7 (July 2008): 881-87.

Buchwald, D., Garrity, D. " Comparison of Patients with Chronic Fatigue Syndrome, Fibromyalgia, and Multiple Chemical Sensitivities." *Archives of Internal Medicine* 154 (1994): 2049-53.

Callender, T.J., Morrow, L., Submaranium, K. "Evaluation of Chronic Neurological Sequelae After Acute Pesticide Poisoning Using Brain SPECT Scans." *Journal of Toxicology and Environmental Health* 41 (1994): 275-84.

Caress, S., Steinemann, A. "A National Population Study of the Prevalence of Multiple Chemical Sensitivity." *Archives of Environmental Health* 59, no. 6 (June 2004): 300-305.

Caress, S., Steinemann, A. "National Prevalence of Asthma and Chemical Hypersensitivity: An Examination of Potential Overlap." *Journal of Occupational and Environmental Medicine* 47, no. 5 (May 2005): 518-22.

Caress, S., Steinemann, A. "A Review of a Two-Phase Population Study of Multiple Chemical Sensitivities. *Environmental Health Perspectives* 111, no. 12 (2003): 1490-97.

Caress, S., Steinemann, A., Waddick, C. "Symptomatology and Etiology of Multiple Chemical Sensitivities in the Southeastern United States." *Archives of Environmental Health: An International Journal* 57, no. 5 (2002): 429-36.

Cone, J., Sult, T. "Acquired Intolerance to Solvents Following Pesticide/ Solvent Exposure in a Building: A New Group of Workers at Risk for Multiple Chemical Sensitivity." *Toxicology and Industrial Health* 8, no. 4 (1992): 29-39.

Costa, L., Li, W., Richter, R., Shih, D., Lusis, A., Furlong, C. "The Role of Paraoxonase (PON1) in the Detoxication of Organophosphates and Its Human Polymorphism. *Chemico-Biological Interactions* 119-20 (1999): 429-38.

Cowan, J., Sinton, C.M., Varley, A.W., Wians, F.H., Haley, R.W., Munford, R.S. "Gene Therapy to Prevent Organophosphate Intoxication." *Toxicology and Applied Pharmacology* 173, no. 1 (May 15, 2001): 16.

Cullen, M.R. "The Worker with Multiple Chemical Sensitivities: An Overview." *Occupational Medicine* 2 (1987): 655-68.

Cullen, M., Pace, P., Redlich, C. "The Experience of the Yale Occupational and Environmental Medicine Clinic with Multiple Chemical Sensitivities," 1986-1991. *Toxicology and Industrial Health* 8 (1992): 15–19.

Davidoff, A., Fogarty, L. "Psychogenic Origins of Multiple Chemical Sensitivity Syndrome: A Critical Review of the Research Literature." *Archives of Environmental Health* 49, no. 5 (1994): 316-25.

Davidoff, A., Keyl, P. "Symptoms and Health Status in Individuals with Multiple Chemical Sensitivities Syndrome from Four Reported Sensitizing Exposures and a General Population Comparison Group." *Archives of Environmental Health* 51, no. 3 (1996): 201-13.

Davidoff, A.L., Meggs, W. "Development of Multiple Chemical Sensitivities in Laborers After Acute Gasoline Fume Exposure in an Underground Tunneling Operation." *Archives of Environmental Health* 53, no. 3 (1998): 183-89.

Doty, R., Deems, D., Frye, R., Pelberg, R., Shapiro, A. "Olfactory Sensitivity, Nasal Resistance, and Autonomic Function in Patients with Multiple Chemical Sensitivities." *Archives of Otolaryngology—Head and Neck Surgery* 114 (1988): 1422-27.

Elberling, J., Dirksen, A., Johansen, J.D., Mosbech, H. "The Capsaicin Cough Reflex in Eczema Patients with Respiratory Symptoms Elicited by Perfume." *Contact Dermatitis* 54, no. 3 (March 2006): 158-64.

Fernandez, M., Bell, I., Schwartz, G. "EEG Sensitization During Chemical Exposure in Women with and Without Chemical Sensitivity of Unknown Etiology." *Toxicology and Industrial Health* 15, nos. 3-4 (1999): 305-12.

Fernández-Solà, J., Liuís Padierna, M., Nogué Xarau, S., Munné, P. "Chronic Fatigue Syndrome and Multiple Chemical Hypersensitivity After Insecticide Exposure." *Medicina Clinica (Barcelona)* 134, no. 12 (April 2, 2005): 451-53.

Fiedler, N., Kipen, H., Natelson, B., Ottenweller, J. "Chemical Sensitivities and the Gulf War." Department of Veterans Affairs Research Center in Basic and Clinical Science Studies of Environmental Hazards. *Regulatory Toxicology and Pharmacology* 24 (1996): S129-S138.

Fincher, E.F., Chang, T.S., Harrell, E.H., Kettkecut, M.C., Rea, W.J., Johnson, A.R., Hickey, H.C., Simon, T.R. "Comparison of Single Photon Computed Tomography Findings in Cases of Healthy Adults and Solvent-Exposed Adults." *American Journal of Industrial Medicine* 31 (1997): 4-14.

Fukuyama, T., Ueda, H., Hayashi, K. Tajima, Y., Shuto, Y., Saito, T.R., Harada, T., Kosaka, T. "Detection of Low-Level Environmental Chemical Allergy by a Long-term Sensitization Method." *Toxicological Letters* 180, no. 1 (July 30, 2008): 1-8.

Galland, L. "Biochemical Abnormalities in Patients with Multiple Chemical Sensitivities." *Occupational Medicine* 2, no. 4 (October-December 1987): 713-20.

Gordon, B.R. "Approaches to Testing for Food and Chemical Sensitivities." *Otolaryngology Clinics of North America* 36, no. 5 (October 2003): 917-40.

Haley, R., Billecke, S., La Du, B. "Association of Low PON1 Type Q (Type A) Arylesterase Activity with Neurologic Symptom Complexes in Gulf War Veterans." *Toxicology and Applied Pharmacology* 157, no. 3(1999): 227-33.

Hasegawa, M., Ohtomo, M., Mita, H., Akiyama, K. "Clinical Aspects of Patients with MCS from the Standpoint of Allergy." *Japanese Journal of Allergology* 54, no. 5 (May 2005): 478-84.

Heuser, G. "Diagnostic Markers in Clinical Immunotoxicology and Neurotoxicology." Editorial. *Journal of Occupational Medicine and Toxicology* 1, no. 4 (1992): v-x.

Heuser, G., Mena, I., Alamous, F. "Neurospect Findings in Patients Exposed to Neurotoxic Chemicals." *Toxicology and Industrial Health* 10, nos. 4-5(1994): 461-571.

Heuser, G., Mena, I. "Neurospect in Neurotoxic Chemical Exposure. Demonstration of Long-Term Functional Abnormalities." *Toxicology and Industrial Health* 14, no. 6 (1998): 813-27.

Heuser, G., Wu, J.C. "Deep Subcortical (Including Limbic) Hypermetabolism in Patients with Chemical Intolerance: Human PET Studies." *Annals of the New York Academy of Sciences* 933 (March 2001): 319-22.

Hojo, S., Ishikawa, S., Kumano, H., Miyata, M., Sakabe, K. "Clinical Characteristics of Physician-Diagnosed Patients with Multiple Chemical Sensitivity in Japan." *International Journal of Hygiene and Environmental Health* 211, nos. 5-6 (October 2008): 682-89.

Inomata, N., Osuna, H., Fujita, H., Ogawa, T. Ikezawa, Z. "Multiple Chemical Sensitivities Following Intolerance to Azo Dye in Sweets in a 5-Year-Old Girl." *Allergology International* 55, no. 2 (June 2006): 203-5.

Ionescu, G., Merk, M., Bradford, R. "Simple Chemiluminesence Assays for Free Radicals in Venous Blood and Serum Samples: Results in Atopic, Psoriasis, MCS and Cancer Patients." *Forsch Komplementarmed* 6, no. 6 (December 1999): 294-300.

Ishibashi, M., Tonori, H., Miki, T., Miyajima, E., Kudo, Y., Tsumoda, M. Sakabe, K., Aizawa, Y. "Classification of Patients Complaining of Sick House Syndrome and/or Multiple Chemical Sensitivity." *Tohoku Journal of Experimental Medicine* 211, no. 3 (March 2007): 223-33.

Jinno, H., Tanaka-Kagawa, T., Obama, T., Miyagawa, M., Yoshikawa, J., Komatsu, K., Tokunaga, H. "Impact of Air Fresheners and Deodorizers on the Indoor Total Volatile Organic Compounds." *Kokuritsu Iyakuhin Shokuhin Eisei Kenkyusho Hokoku* 125 (2007): 72-78.

Kailen, E.W., Brooks, C.R. "Systemic Toxic Reactions to Soft Plastic Food Containers." *Medical Annals of D.C.* 32 (1963): 1-8.

Kilburn K. "Effects of Diesel Exhaust on Neurobehavioral and Pulmonary Functions." *Archives of Environmental Health* 55, no. 1 (January/February 2000).

Kimata, H. "Effect of Exposure to Volatile Organic compounds on Plasma Levels of Neuropeptides, Nerve Growth Factor and Histamine in Patients with Self-Reported Multiple Chemical Sensitivity." *International Journal of Hygiene and Environmental Health* 207, no. 2 (February 2004): 159-63.

Kimata, H. "Exposure to Road Traffic Enhances Allergic Skin Wheal Responses and Increases Plasma Neuropeptides and Neurotrophins in Patients with Atopic Eczema/Dermatitis Syndrome." *International Journal of Hygiene and Environmental Health* 207, no. 1 (January 2004): 45-49.

Kipen, H.M., Hallman, W., Kang, H., Fiedler, N., Natelson, B.H. "Prevalence of Chronic Fatigue and Chemical Sensitivities in Gulf Registry

Veterans." *Archives of Environmental Health* 54, no. 5 (September-October 1999): 309-11.

Kruetzer, R., Neutra, R., Lashuay, N. "Prevalence of People Reporting Sensitivities to Chemicals in a Population-Based Survey." *American Journal of Epidemiology* 150, no. 1 (1999): 1-12.

Lax, M., Henneberger, P. "Patients with Multiple Chemical Sensitivities in an Occupational Health Clinic: Presentation and Follow-up." *Archives of Environmental Health* 50, no. 6 (1995): 425-31.

Lee, T.G. "Health Symptoms Caused by Molds in a Courthouse." *Archives of Environmental Health* 58, no. 7 (July 2003): 442-46.

Levallois, P., Neutra, R., Lee, G., Hristoa, L. "Study of Self-Reported Hypersensitivity to Electromagnetic Fields in California." *Environmental Health Perspectives* 110, Supplement 4 (August 2002): 619-23.

Lieberman, A.D., Craven, M.R. "Reactive Intestinal Dysfunction Syndrome (RIDS) Caused by Chemical Exposures." *Archives of Environmental Health* 54, no. 5 (September-October 1999): 365-66.

McFadden, S. "Phenotype Variation in Xenobiotic Metabolism and Adverse Environmental Response: Focus on Sulfur-Dependant Detoxification Pathways." *Toxicology* 111 (1996): 43-65.

McKeown-Eyssen, G., Baines, C., Cole, D.E., Riley, N. Tyndale, R.F., Marshall, L, Jazmaji, V. "Case-Control Study of Genotypes in Multiple Chemical Sensitivity: CYP2D6, NAT1, NAT2, PON1, PON2 AND MTHFR." *International Journal of Epidemiology* (July 15, 2004).

Meggs, W.J. "Hypothesis for Induction and Propagation of Chemical Sensitivity Based on Biopsy Studies." Review. *Environmental Health Perspectives* 105 (March 1997).

Meggs, W.J. "Neurogenic Switching: A Hypothesis for a Mechanism for Shifting the Site of Inflammation in Allergy and Chemical Sensitivity." *Environmental Health Perspectives* 103, no. 1 (January 1995): 54-56.

Meggs, W. "RADS and RUDS—The Toxic Induction of Asthma and Rhinitis." *Clinical Toxicology* 32, no. 5 (1994): 487-501.

Meggs, W., Cleveland, C. "Rhinolaryngoscopic Examination of Patients with the Multiple Chemical Sensitivity Syndrome." *Archives of Environmental Health* 41, no. 1 (1993): 14-18.

Meggs, W., Dunn, K., Bloch, R., Goodman, P., Davidoff, L. "Prevalence and Nature of Allergy and Chemical Sensitivity in a General Population." *Archives of Environmental Health* 51, no. 4 (1996): 275-82.

Meggs, W.J., Elsheik, T., Metzger, W.J., Albernaz, M., Bloch, R.M. "Nasal Pathology and Ultrastructure in Patients with Chronic Airway Inflammation Following an Irritant Exposure." *Journal of Toxicology-Clinical Toxicology* 34, no. 4 (1996): 383-96.

Migliore, A., Bizzi, E., Massafra, U., Capuano, A., Martin, L.S. "Multiple Chemical Sensitivity Syndrome in Sjögren's Syndrome Patients: Casual Association or Related Diseases?" *Archives of Environmental and Occupational Health* 61, no. 6 (November-December 2006): 285-87.

Miller, C.S. "Possible Models for Multiple Chemical Sensitivity: Conceptual Issues and Role of the Limbic System. Advancing the Understanding of Multiple Chemical Sensitivity." Association of Occupational and Environmental Clinics. *Toxicology and Industrial Health* 8, no. 4 (1992): 181-202.

Miller, C.S. "White Paper: Chemical Sensitivity: History and Phenomenology." *Toxicology and Industrial Health* 10, no. 4-5 (1994): 253-76.

Miller, C.S., Gammage, R.B., Jankovic, J.T. " Exacerbation of Chemical Sensitivity: A Case Study." *Toxicology and Industrial Health* 15, nos. 3-4 (April-June 1999): 398-402.

Miller, C., Mitzel, H. "Chemical Sensitivity Attributed to Pesticide Exposure Versus Remodeling." *Archives of Environmental Health* 50, no. 2 (1995): 119.

Miller, C. "Toxicant-Induced Loss of Tolerance: An Emerging Theory of Disease?" *Environmental Health Perspectives* 105, Supplement 2 (1997): 445-53.

Miller, C., Prihoda, T. "The Environmental Exposure and Sensitivity Inventory (EESI): A Standardized Approach for Measuring Chemical Intolerances for Research and Applications." *Toxicology and Industrial Health* 15 (1999): 370-85.

Miller, C., Prihoda, T. "A Controlled Comparison of Symptoms and Chemical Intolerances Reported by Gulf War Veterans, Implant Recipients, and Persons with Multiple Chemical Sensitivity." *Toxicology and Industrial Health* 15 (1999): 386-97.

Miller, C., Ashford, N., Doty, R., Lamielle, M., Otto, D., Rahill, A., Wallace, L. "Empirical Approaches for the Investigation of Toxicant-Induced Loss of Tolerance." *Environmental Health Perspectives* 105, Supplement 2 (1997): 515-19.

Miller, C., Gammage, R., Jankovic, J. "Exacerbation of Chemical Sensitivity: A Case Study." *Toxicology and Industrial Health* 15 (1999): 398-402.

Millqvist, E., Bengtsson, U., Lowhagen, O. "Provocations with Perfume in the Eyes Induce Airway Symptoms in Patients with Sensory Hyper-reactivity." *Allergy* 54, no. 5 (May 1999): 495-99.

Millqvist, E., Ternesten-Hasséus, E., Ståhl, A., Bende, M. "Changes in Levels of Nerve Growth Factor in Nasal Secretions after Capsaicin Inhalation in Patients with Airway Symptoms from Scents and Chemicals." *Environmental Health Perspectives* 113, no. 7 (July 2005): 849-52.

Nethercott, J., Davidoff, L., Curbow, B., Abbey, H. "Multiple Chemical Sensitivities Syndrome: Toward a Working Case Definition." *Archives of Environmental Health* 48 (1993): 19-26.

Nogué, S., Fernández-Solá, J., Rovira, E., Montori, E., Fernández-Huerta, J.M., Munné, P. "Multiple Chemical Sensitivity: Study of 52 Cases." *Medicina Clinica (Barcelona)* 129, no. 3 (June 16, 2007): 96-98.

Overstreet, D.H., Djuric, V. "A Genetic Rat Model of Cholinergic Hypersensitivity: Implications for Chemical Intolerance, Chronic Fatigue, and Asthma." *Annals of the New York Academy of Science* 933 (March 2001): 92-102.

Overstreet, D., Miller, C., Janowsky, D., Russell, R. "Potential Animal Model of Multiple Chemical Sensitivity with Cholinergic Supersensitivity." *Toxicology* 111 (1996): 119-34.

Pall, M.L. "Elevated Nitric Oxide-Peroxynitrite Theory of Multiple Chemical Sensitivity: Central Role of N-Methyl-D-Aspartate Receptors in the Sensitivity Mechanism." *Environmental Health Perspectives* 111, no. 12 (September 2003): 1461-64.

Randolph, T.G. "Clinical Manifestations of Individual Susceptibility to Insecticides and Related Materials." *Industrial Medicine and Surgery* 34 (February 1965): 134-42.

Randolph, T.G. "Dynamics, Diagnosis, and Treatment of Food Allergy." Review. *Otolaryngology Clinics of North America* 7, no. 3 (October 1974): 617-35.

Randolph, T.G. "Ecologic Orientation in Medicine: Comprehensive Environmental Control in Diagnosis and Therapy." *Annals of Allergy* 23 (January 1965): 7-22.

Randolph, T.G. "Human Ecology and Susceptibility to the Chemical Environment." *Annals of Allergy* 19 (May 1961): 518-40.

Randolph, T.G. "Human Ecology and Susceptibility to the Chemical Environment: Air Pollution." *Annals of Allergy* 19 (June 1961): 657-77.

Randolph, T.G. "Human Ecology and Susceptibility to the Chemical Environment." *Annals of Allergy.* 19 (July 1961): 779-99.

Randolph, T.G. "Human Ecology and Susceptibility to the Chemical Environment." *Annals of Allergy.* 19 (August 1961): 908-29.

Rea, W.J. "Environmentally Triggered Cardiac Disease." *Annals of Allergy* 40 (April 1978): 243-51.

Rea, W.J. "Environmentally Triggered Small Vessel Vasculitis." *Annals of Allergy* 38 (April 1977): 245-51.

Rea, W.J. "Environmentally Triggered Thrombophlebitis." *Annals of Allergy* 37, no. 2 (August 1976): 101-9.

Rea, W.J., Peters, D.W., Smiley, R.E., Edgar, R., Greenberg, M., Fenyves, E. "Recurrent Environmentally Triggered Thrombophlebitis: A Five-Year Follow-up." *Annals of Allergy* 47, no. 5, pt. 1 (November 1981): 338-44.

Rogers, W.R., Miller, C.S., Bunegin, L "A Rat Model of Neurobehavioral Sensitization to Toluene." *Toxicology and Industrial Health* 15, nos. 3-4 (April-June 1999): 356-69.

Ross, G.H. "Clinical Characteristics of Chemical Sensitivity: An Illustrative Case History of Asthma and MCS." *Environmental Health Perspectives* 105, Supplement 2 (March 1997): 437-41.

Ross, G.H. "History and Clinical Presentation of the Chemically Sensitive Patient." *Toxicology and Industrial Health* 8, no. 4 (July-August 1992): 21-28.

Ross, G.H., Rea, W.J., Johnson, A.R., Hickey, D.C., Simon, T.R. "Neurotoxicity in Single Photon Computed Tomography Brain Scans of Patients Reporting Chemical Sensitivities." *Toxicology and Industrial Health* 15 (1999): 415-20.

Rossi, J. "Sensitization Induced by Kindling and Kindling-Related Phenomena as a Model for Multiple Chemical Sensitivity." *Toxicology* 111, nos. 1-3 (July 17, 1996): 87-100.

Shirakawa, S., Ishikawa, S., Miyata, M., Rea, W.J., Johnson, A.R. "A Pupillographical Study on the Presence of Organochlorine Pesticides in Autonomic Nerve Disturbance." *Nippon Ganka Gakkai Zasshi* 94, no. 4 (April 1990): 418-23.

Simon, T.R., Hicket, D.C., Fincher, C.E., Johnson, A.R., Ross, G.H. and Rea, W.J. "Single Photon Computed Tomography of the Brain in Patients with Chemical Sensitivities." *Toxicology and Industrial Health* 10, nos. 4-5 (1994): 573-77.

Simon, T.R., Rea, W.J. "Use of Functional Brian Imaging in the Evaluation of Exposure to Mycotoxins and Toxins Encountered in Desert Storm/Desert Shield." *Archives of Environmental Health* 58, no. 7 (July 2003): 406-9.

Sorg, B.A., Hochstatter, T. "Behavioral Sensitization After Repeated Formaldehyde Exposure in Rats." *Toxicology and Industrial Health* 15, nos. 3-4 (April-June 1999): 346-55.

Sorg, B.A. "Multiple Chemical Sensitivity: Potential Role for Neural-sensitization." Review. *Critical Reviews in Neurobiology* 13, no. 3 (1999): 283-316.

Sorg B. "Proposed Animal Model for Multiple Chemical Sensitivity in Studies with Formalin." *Toxicology* 111(1996): 135-45.

Spencer, T.R., Schur, P.M. "The Challenge of Multiple Chemical Sensitivity." *Journal of Environmental Health* 70, no. 10 (June 2008): 24-27.

Steinemann, A. "Fragranced Consumer Products and Undisclosed Ingredients." *Environmental Impact Assessment Review.* Online publication, July 23, 2008. Forthcoming in journal.

Stephens, R., Spurgeon, A., Calvert, I., et al. " Neuropsychological Effect of Long-Term Exposure to Organophosphates in Sheep Dip." *Lancet* 3459 (1995): 1135-39.

Ternesten-Hasseus, E., Bende, M., Millqvist, E. "Increased Capsaicin Cough Sensitivity in Patients with Multiple Chemical Sensitivity." *Journal of Occupational and Environmental Medicine* 44, no. 11 (November 2002).

Thrasher, J.D., Heuser, G., Broughton, A. "Immunological Abnormalities in Humans Chronically Exposed to Chlorpyrifos." *Archives of Environmental Health* 57, no. 3 (May-June 2002): 181-87.

Thrasher, J.D., Vojdani, A., Cheung, G., Heuser, G. "Evidence for Formaldehyde Antibodies and Altered Cellular Immunity in Subjects Exposed to Formaldehyde in Mobile Homes." *Archives of Environmental Health* 42, no. 6 (November-December 1987): 347-50.

Welch, L.S., Sokas, R. "Development of Multiple Chemical Sensitivity After an Outbreak of Sick-Building Syndrome." *Toxicology and Industrial Health* 8, no. 4 (1991): 47-65.

Wiesmuller, G.A., et al. "Nasal Function in Self-Reported Chemically Intolerant Individuals." *Archives of Environmental Health* 57, no. 3 (May-June 2002): 247-54.

Ziem, G.E. "Multiple Chemical Sensitivity: Treatment and Follow-up with Avoidance and Control of Chemical Exposures. Advancing the Understanding of Multiple Chemical Sensitivity." Association of Occupational and Environmental Clinics. *Toxicology and Industrial Health* 8, no. 4 (1992): 181-202.

Ziem., G.E., McTamney, J. "Profile of Patients with Chemical Injury and Sensitivity." *Environmental Health Perspectives* 105, Supplement 2 (March 1997): 417-36.

Index